PRESCRIPTION FOR LEARNING

Techniques, games
and activities

Ruth Chambers
Gill Wakley
Zafar Iqbal
and
Steve Field

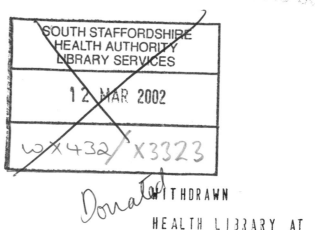
Radcliffe Medical Press

Radcliffe Medical Press Ltd
18 Marcham Road
Abingdon
Oxon OX14 1AA
United Kingdom

www.radcliffe-oxford.com
The Radcliffe Medical Press electronic catalogue and online ordering facility.
Direct sales to anywhere in the world.

British Library Cataloguing in Publication Data

A catalogue record for this book is available from the British Library.

ISBN 1 85775 530 8

Typeset by Advance Typesetting Ltd, Oxfordshire
Printed and bound by TJ International Ltd, Padstow, Cornwall

Contents

About the authors

Ruth Chambers BM BS, BMed Sci, DRCOG, Cert Med Ed, DM, FRCGP has been a GP for 22 years and is currently the professor of primary care development at Staffordshire University. Ruth has designed and organised many types of educational initiatives, including distance-learning programmes. Recently she has developed a keen interest in working with GPs, nurses and others in primary care on clinical governance and practice personal and professional development plans. She has co-authored a series of books designed to help readers to draw up their own personal development plans or practice learning plans on important clinical topics.

Gill Wakley MB ChB, MFFP, MIPM, MD started in general practice in 1966, but transferred to community medicine shortly afterwards and then into public health. A desire for increased contact with patients caused a move back into general practice, together with community gynaecology, in 1978. She has been combining the two in varying amounts ever since. Throughout Gill has been heavily involved in learning and teaching. She was in a training general practice, became an instructing doctor and a regional assessor in family planning, and was until recently a senior clinical lecturer in the Primary Care Department at Keele University. Like Ruth, she has run all types of educational initiatives and activities, from individual mentoring and instruction to small group work, plenary lectures, distance-learning programmes, workshops and courses for a wide range of health professionals and lay people.

Zafar Iqbal MB BS, DCH, MRCGP, FFPHM entered public health medicine after completing a general practice vocational training scheme in 1989. He became a public health consultant at South Staffordshire Health Authority in 1994, and is also currently an honorary senior lecturer in public health medicine at Birmingham University. Zafar is a member of the regional training executive committee for public health medicine, and is a faculty visitor for regional public health training programmes. In the last few years he has recommenced his career in general practice on a sessional basis.

Zafar has recently been involved in a variety of initiatives to promote a more systematic approach to the management of coronary heart disease in the primary care setting. His other main interest is clinical governance and the way in which this links in with delivering the National Service Frameworks.

Steve Field MB ChB, DRCOG, MMEd, FRCGP is acting regional postgraduate dean for the West Midlands. He was formerly director of postgraduate general practice education. He is vice-chair of the Committee of GP Education Directors (COGPED), chair of the Implementation Committee for the new UK GP Registrar Scheme and chair of the National Summative Assessment Board for General Practice. He has been a GP since 1986, and is a GP principal in inner-city Birmingham. He is an MRCGP examiner, a member of the Royal College of General Practitioners' examination board and chair of the RCGP's education network.

Steve continues to be actively involved in teaching and learning, and has a particular interest in communication skills and assessment methodologies.

Acknowledgements

Some of the games, activities and techniques that are described in this book are adapted from those we have gleaned from colleagues and teachers over the years. We should like to thank them and acknowledge their contributions. We have not knowingly reproduced any unmodified exercises without acknowledging the source.

List of games, activities and learning techniques

Many of these exercises can be adapted to teach topics or approaches to learning other than those on which they are focused in this book. Use them and adapt them to create your own learning activities in your own field.

1

Introduction: why you need games, activities and learning techniques

This book presents a wide variety of games, activities and techniques that a teacher or tutor can use to help others to learn. Learning is most powerful when it is both hard work and fun. This usually means that it is interactive and based on experience – challenging but at the same time possible.

Each chapter has a short introduction to the topic followed by several exercises that are mainly interactive and designed to reinforce learning in any of the three domains of knowledge, skills and attitudes. These will not only make teaching more interesting, but will provide developmental opportunities for individuals and teams of learners to benefit much more from the learning events. At the same time they are encouraged to apply what they learn in their own settings.

The games, activities and learning techniques are drawn from a variety of sources, including our own experience. Some are donated by other educators, others are well-known games adulterated by us for new uses, and yet others have been created by us for this book. We or others have tried and tested all of the exercises on a variety of audiences.

There is an evolving culture of a 'learning environment' in the health service. Much of what has to be learned is about attitudes and feelings rather than simply knowledge and skills. Traditional types of education (e.g. in the lecture theatre) are inappropriate for teaching about attitudes and feelings. There will be more emphasis on learning in teams in-house. Teams that are novices to this way of learning may need some help in getting started with self-directed learning, but be unable to afford a facilitator. Exercises and activities should help them to start and sustain a more effective educational event. Such a session should be more enjoyable, encourage teambuilding, and be more likely to be repeated.

We know that the most successful learning:[1]

- is based on what is already known by the learner
- is led by the learner's own identified needs

- involves active participation by the learner
- uses the learner's own resources
- includes relevant and timely feedback
- includes self-assessment.

The different games, activities and techniques included here are relevant to one or more of these criteria for successful learning. Some of them build on the learner's previous experience and others aid learners in identifying areas of ignorance of which they were previously unaware. All of the activities require participants to interact with the teacher or facilitator and usually each other, thereby reinforcing the learning of the session. Most of the activities we describe in this book enable the learner to self-assess their performance and receive feedback from peers about how they are doing.

Box 1.1:

A *teacher* does not just need sufficient knowledge, skills and resources, but also the right attitudes and understanding of the overall context and cultural environment to be able to make the teaching relevant to the learner's needs. Choose from the wealth of games, activities and techniques described here those that are relevant to the individuals whom you teach and appropriate for their circumstances or the learning event.

No single method of teaching is the best one. Different methods suit different situations and different learners and teachers. Most people learn best by 'doing' – using active methods of learning rather than sitting passively in a lecture theatre listening to a series of keynote lectures. An ancient Chinese proverb makes exactly this point:

I hear and I forget
I see and I remember
I do and I understand.

You should know and be able to employ a variety of active educational methods and choose the methods you use carefully to fit in best with what you are trying to teach or learn about.
    A good teacher should:

- stimulate the learner
- challenge the learner
- interest the learner
- involve the learner
- prepare well so that the context and content are clear and focused
- encourage the learner – with positive feedback

- understand the learner's needs
- have an appropriate plan to meet the learner's needs
- use a style of delivery that suits the learner's needs
- evaluate both the teaching and the learning
- refine future teaching in the light of this evaluation
- be a lifelong learner.

The games, activities and learning techniques included here will help you to deliver your teaching so that your 'students' describe you as a 'good teacher'.

Learning styles

Everyone has their own preferred learning style(s). This means that there may be a mismatch between the teacher's preferred style and those of the individuals he or she is addressing. Therefore it is important that teachers are aware of their own preferences and how these might enrapture or bore people with other learning styles. The games, activities and learning techniques in this book should enable teachers to vary their style and mode of delivery in a single teaching session, so that there is something of interest for everyone.

Honey and Mumford have described four learning styles:[2]

1   *Activists*: like to be fully involved in new experiences, are open-minded, will try anything once, and thrive on the challenge of new experiences but soon get bored and want to go on to the next challenge. They are gregarious and like to be the centre of attention.

Activists learn best through new experiences, short activities, and situations where they can occupy centre stage (e.g. chairing meetings, leading discussions), when allowed to generate new ideas and have a go at things or brainstorm ideas.

2   *Reflectors*: like to stand back, think about things thoroughly and obtain plenty of information before reaching a conclusion. They are cautious, take a back seat in meetings and discussions, adopt a low profile and appear tolerant and unruffled. When they do act it is by using the wide picture of their own and others' views.

Reflectors learn best from situations where they are allowed to watch and think about activities before acting. They conduct research first of all, review the evidence, produce carefully constructed reports and can reach decisions in their own time.

3   *Theorists*: like to adapt and integrate observations into logical maps and models using step-by-step processes. They tend to be perfectionists, detached, analytical and objective. They reject anything that is subjective or flippant, or that involves lateral thinking.

Theorists learn best from activities in which there are plans, maps and models to describe what is going on. They prefer to take time to explore the methodology, to work with structured situations with a clear purpose, and to be offered complex situations to understand and be intellectually stretched.

4 *Pragmatists*: like to try out ideas, theories and techniques to see whether they work in practice. They will act quickly and confidently in response to ideas that attract them, and become impatient with ruminating and open-ended discussions. They are down-to-earth people who like solving problems and making practical decisions, responding to problems as a challenge.

Pragmatists learn best when there is an obvious link between the subject and their job. They enjoy trying out techniques involving coaching and feedback, practical issues, having real problems to solve and being given the immediate opportunity to implement what has been learned.

There are several models describing learning styles that can be useful when designing learning opportunities. *Convergent thinkers* tend to find just one solution to a problem, but discussion and training can enable them to learn more divergent thinking skills where new ideas and exploration of ideas are preferred. The skills of *divergent thinkers* are more useful in the real world where there are multiple opportunities.

Serialists learn one step after another, and *holistic thinkers* prefer to look at the whole picture first and then focus on the constituent parts. It is useful to think of this type of model when designing materials that will be used for self-teaching, as the material will need to suit both types of thinker.

Another type of model, that of *deep processors* (who read through something and summarise the main points mentally) and *surface processors* (who skim through something rapidly, trying to remember as much as possible), is useful for informing the development of distance-learning packages.

Barriers to personal learning

McGiveney[3] suggests that reluctance to engage in adult education may have more to do with attitudes, perceptions and expectations than with any physical barriers. She summarises a number of studies that together provide a list of possible reasons for non-participation. The list includes the following:

- perceptions of inappropriateness or lack of relevance
- hostility towards previous learning experiences
- the belief that one is too old to learn
- lack of confidence in one's ability to learn
- lack of awareness of learning needs.

She also comments on the practical difficulties that prevent people from taking up educational opportunities. These include the following:

- lack of time
- lack of money
- transport difficulties
- such opportunities being offered at the wrong time
- childcare difficulties.

She then discusses how these multiple factors combine and interact. Uptake of learning can be improved by removing just one or two major obstacles.

The educational cycle

The educational cycle is a simple and well-understood model in education, and its principles are applicable to many teaching and learning situations within medical and health education.

The four steps in the cycle are as follows:[4]

1 assessing the individual's needs
2 setting educational objectives
3 choosing and using a variety of methods of teaching and learning
4 assessing whether learning has occurred.

The next stage involves going on to determine the next set of objectives and repeating the above process.

Principles of adult learning

Many people talk about adult learning and the fact that many trainees do not behave as adults, but expect to be 'spoon-fed'. However, it is not just a matter of letting trainees or students get on with learning entirely on their own. It is essential that adult learning is *facilitated* by the trainer, and the games, activities and learning techniques described in this book will help any teacher or trainer to facilitate other people's learning.

Brookfield's principles of adult learning state the following.[5]

1 *Participation is voluntary*. The decision to learn is that of the learner.
2 *There should be mutual respect* between teachers and learners, and also among learners.
3 *Collaboration is important*, both between learners and teachers and among learners.
4 *Action and reflection* form a continuous process of investigation, exploration, action, reflection and further action.

5   *Critical reflection* brings awareness that alternatives can be presented as challenges to the learner to gather evidence, ask questions and develop a critically aware frame of mind.
6   *Nurturing of self-directed adults is important.*

Education and training

There is sometimes confusion about the differences between the terms 'education' and 'training'. Often both occur together within a learning experience. The two may be differentiated by thinking of:

*   education as being about doing things better
*   training as being about taking on new tasks.

Being a more effective facilitator, trainer, tutor, motivator and communicator

The games, activities and learning techniques that we include here should help you to enhance your effectiveness in whatever role you are playing – by really engaging with the participants who are learning from you.

How to use the exercises: giving good feedback

Each exercise is broken down to describe the purpose of the activity and how to carry it out. We give you insight into the knowledge, skills and attitudes that you will be trying to influence in the learners. We explain how to make the exercise work well, and caution you about what might go wrong. We have allocated each game, activity or learning technique to the topic of a particular chapter, but as you will see, most can be easily adapted to relay learning about the topics and skills of a number of other chapters.

So how can constructive feedback be given? There is one golden rule – give positive praise of things that have been done well first. Sometimes colleagues launch straight into criticism of faults after an exercise or when reviewing a task at work. They have to be reminded that they must feed back the good points first, and only later discuss points which need improving, in a helpful and constructive way.

Giving feedback constructively using one of the models available will improve the educational climate and the learning outcomes in your organisation, will improve competence and will increase the motivation of those colleagues with whom you work.

The Pendleton model is widely used in the health setting.[6] It is a step-by-step model in which every step is important, and it should be carried out in the order described below.

1 The learner first goes and performs the activity.
2 Questions are allowed only on points of clarification of fact.
3 The learner states what they thought was done well.
4 The teacher states what they thought was done well.
5 The learner states what was not done so well and could be improved upon.
6 The teacher states what was not done so well, and suggests ways to improve this, with discussion conducted in a helpful and constructive manner.

This model is useful for giving and receiving feedback when doing various 'microteaching' exercises on a training course. It does provide a very good structure for giving feedback in a constructive manner.

Another method that comes from the University of Chicago is similar to Pendleton's model, but has the advantage of starting with a reminder of the aims and objectives that the learner should be addressing. It has six steps as described below:[1]

1 Review the aims and objectives of the task at the start.
2 Give interim feedback of a positive nature.
3 Ask the learner to give you their own self-appraisal of their performance.
4 Give feedback focusing on behaviour rather than on personality (e.g. what actually happened, concentrating on the facts and not your opinions).
5 Give specific examples to illustrate your views.
6 Suggest specific strategies for the learner to improve their performance.

Tips for you as a teacher

- Vary the pace and style of your educational sessions using a variety of the games, activities and learning techniques described in this book.
- Consider giving delegates the option of going outside the venue for a walk while doing work in pairs (e.g. after lunch, when most people are likely to feel sleepy).
- Another alternative to organising group work discussion in pairs, trios or larger small groups is to start in pairs for the initial task, then double up to a foursome to exchange the key points of the pairs' discussions and continue with the task, and then double up to an eightsome and repeat the process (this approach is termed a 'snowball').
- Get to the venue early!

- Know the venue. Visit it before the event, check and familiarise yourself with the audiovisual aids, microphones, etc., check that there is an over-head projector, data projector (take your laptop), etc., and find out whether there is an audiovisual technician on hand.
- Consider comfort and safety issues. Dress comfortably, ensure that you tell the participants where the toilets and the fire exits are situated at the start of the meeting, and clarify the time of comfort/coffee and food breaks. Do not go on for too long! Education is more effective if you are comfortable and not desperate to go to the toilet. Make sure that drinks are easily available close to the action, and avoid interruptions (especially bleeps and mobile phones) and put up a sign to keep out non-participants.
- Who are the participants? Before the education session spend some time considering the participants, their background, their possible level of understanding, skill mix, etc.
- Prevent trouble before it happens. Monitor the group dynamics and your 'audience's' body language at all times, and vary the pace or style or intervene appropriately. Take critical comments seriously, and consider whether there is any preventive or restorative action you could take.

Ground rules

Opening impressions have an important bearing on the atmosphere for the rest of the event or the remaining training sessions. Any problems in an initial session may have a lasting effect, whilst a successful start will boost the learning environment in future sessions. Two techniques that can be used to create a successful environment in the initial period include establishing 'ground rules' with the participants, and helping them to get to know each other and settle in through the use of 'ice-breaker' techniques.

It is important to clarify the ground rules, as this helps to create a 'safe' environment. Establishing the ground rules is an excellent way of releasing tension and reducing nervousness, as it allows people to shape the culture and boundaries in which they wish to work.

Common areas encompassed by ground rules include the following:

- ensure confidentiality, particularly when members from the same organisation are present. Nothing heard within the group should be repeated or, if information is given, attributed to a group member without their permission
- encourage mutual respect, allowing all opinions to be heard
- feedback should be constructive and positive, any criticism being helpful and not destructive
- people should be able to opt out of certain exercises. The group may wish to set criteria for how and when this could happen (e.g. whether

an explanation is offered to the facilitator or to the group, or is required at all)

- give each other permission to take 'time out' or a break if a participant is finding a subject emotionally threatening (e.g. if a relative has recently died or if they have been diagnosed with a particular illness, etc.)
- limit interruptions from personal business (e.g. turn off mobile phones, ask individuals to fix other appointments outside the group's meeting times or course timetable)
- be punctual
- do not smoke at the meeting or event, or in the group's vicinity.

The facilitator should allow participants to modify these ground rules by group consensus at any stage during the series of learning events or workshop (*see* Exercise 6.1 for an exercise concerned with the setting of ground rules).

References

1 Roland M, Holden J and Campbell S (1999) *Quality Assessment for General Practice: supporting clinical governance in primary care groups.* National Primary Care Research and Development Centre, University of Manchester, Manchester.

2 Honey P and Mumford A (1986) *Using Your Learning Styles*. Peter Honey, Maidenhead.

3 McGiveney V (1990) *Education's for Other People: access to education for non-participant adults. Section 1*. National Institute for the Advancement of Community Education, Leicester.

4 Chambers R and Wall D (2000) *Teaching Made Easy*. Radcliffe Medical Press, Oxford.

5 Brookfield SD (1986) *Understanding and Facilitating Adult Learning*. Open University Press, Milton Keynes.

6 Pendleton D, Schofield T, Tate P and Havelock P (1984) *The Consultation: an approach to teaching and learning*. Oxford Medical Publications, Oxford.

Much of the material in this chapter is derived from Chambers R and Wall D (2000) *Teaching Made Easy*. Radcliffe Medical Press, Oxford.

Games, activities and learning techniques

Unlike the 60 or so exercises in the other chapters, those included in Chapter 1 are described only briefly. They are simple checklists or learning activities that do not warrant in-depth instructions or insight into the way in which they work in practice, in contrast to the detailed exercises in the rest of the book.

Exercise 1.1 Put together a toolkit

Put together your own toolkit to take along to any situations where you are teaching, giving a presentation or organising a learning event, so that you are prepared for anything.

Pack the following:

- 'Post-it' notes for anonymised input and brainstorming
- Blu-Tack
- spare flip-chart pens of various colours/whiteboard pens
- a timer for pacing the event (this might be a humorous timer such as a cock or a pig from a kitchenware shop)
- a bell to call delegates in from lunch or from outside the venue if they are walking or smoking there
- flags or a traffic-light system of some kind (e.g. red, amber and green cards) to indicate discreetly to speakers or participants who are giving presentations when their time is up
- comments cards so that participants can write messages or reminders as they swap information or request copies of your material or that of other participants
- spare A4 paper – participants often forget to bring any with them
- new overhead-projector transparencies for small groups to prepare feedback presentations if appropriate
- several old Sunday newspapers – you might want to cut them up for various exercises
- your diary to prompt students about future meetings
- a small screwdriver – just in case
- tissues or kitchen roll to clean the lens of the overhead projector and mop up any spilt water or coffee
- a spare extension lead with at least two sockets – invaluable for rooms where the sockets are nowhere near the place where you want to put the projector, etc.
- coins or a ruler to pin down the curling edges of transparencies
- rubber bands to hold papers, pencils or files together
- a spare overhead-projector bulb
- a calculator – you may need this for tallying the scores in the various exercises.

Exercise 1.2 How to run the most marvellous workshop

At the start of a workshop, the participants are uncertain and may have mixed feelings and views about being there at all. There may be:

- a lack of rapport between individuals
- group inertia
- apprehension and nervousness
- a sense of not knowing what to expect
- anticipation
- a range of feelings, from excitement and enthusiasm to hostility or apathy
- a mix of some people with clear learning goals and others who believe that the event is timewasting
- relief and pleasure at being able to get away from everyday work.

1   Plan the workshop well in advance.
2   Check the venue before you book it. Make sure that it is:
   - the right size (neither too large nor or too small)
   - comfortable (not smelly, dirty, too hot or too noisy)
   - properly equipped for your needs (e.g. with tables, chairs, overhead projector, projector, electric sockets, blackout, flip chart, etc.)
   - suitable for the participants (e.g. with toilet facilities in sufficient numbers for the gender of the expected delegates, premises accessible to people with physical handicaps, etc.)
   - provided with facilities for refreshments or food suitable for the time of day and for the participants
   - easily found by the participants – send a map *and* directions, and signpost the venue if possible.
3   Make sure that the target participants know about the workshop in plenty of time to arrange their diaries.
4   Check that the right date and time appear on any advertising material.
5   Advertise the start and finish and a draft of the programme, so that people have some idea of what to expect.
6   Prepare a more detailed programme when you know who is presenting/attending, but be prepared to modify it in response to feedback from the participants.
7   Have long enough breaks for people to have drinks and go to the toilet, especially if these facilities are some distance from the meeting rooms.
8   Make sure that everyone feels welcome and part of the group.
9   Introduce yourself and give the participants an opportunity to introduce themselves.

10   Make sure that people know the aims of the workshop (both yours and theirs).

11   Start on time (unless there is an acceptable reason for a late start, such as no one having arrived because of fog!).

12   Go to breaks on time, so that no one is too hungry, thirsty or uncomfortable to learn.

13   Finish on time.

14   Encourage everyone to participate by varying the type of activity to suit different types of learners and people who find speaking in a large group intimidating.

15   Restrain yourself from talking too much or organising adult learners as if they were children or incompetent.

16   Look after yourself, so that you are in the best state to run the workshop well.

Add to the above list yourself, and use it as a checklist.

Exercise 1.3   Some 'ice-breakers'

The appropriate exercise should be selected to literally 'break the ice' at the beginning of the workshop. Ice-breakers need to be quick (10–30 minutes), fun, develop rapport and encourage remembering of names.

1   Participants pair up and introduce themselves to each other, swapping two or three interesting facts about themselves. They then turn to the rest of the group, and one of the pair introduces the other to the main group. A soft ball is then thrown from person to person. However, before a ball can be thrown, the name and facts of the intended recipient should be called out by the person throwing the ball. This exercise can be repeated at the beginning of each session until the participants are familiar with each others' names. The ice-breaker finishes when everyone has received the ball.

2   The facilitator prepares a slightly different list of unusual characteristics of the participants on cards and hands them out to each member of the group. This list could include, for example, a person with ladies shoe size 3, someone who has hitched a lift on the motorway, someone who has an arts degree, someone who has been to South America, someone who has played in a rock band, someone who has ridden a Harley Davidson motorbike, someone who has three children, etc. The number of items needs to be greater than the number of people in the group. Individuals are asked to mingle and introduce themselves to people, and to tick off characteristics as they come across people with them. An element of competition

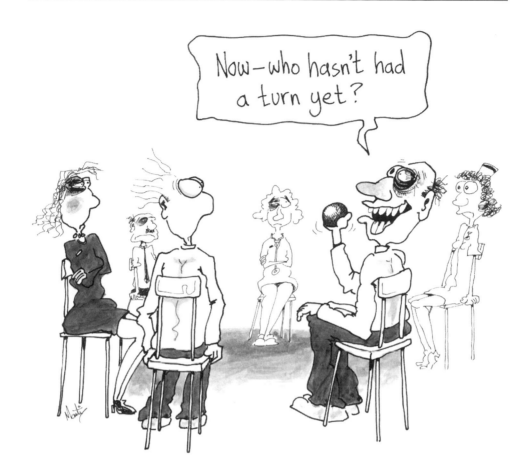

can be introduced, with the winner being the person who finds the most matches.

You will find other 'ice-breaker' exercises in the book at the end of various chapters (e.g. Exercises 4.1 and 4.3 in Chapter 4 on communication).

Exercise 1.4 An 'energiser'

There will be times during the day, particularly after lunch, when both mental and physical fatigue sets in. Energisers can be used to stimulate group dynamics and shake people out of lethargy. One example will be given here.

Participants are divided into small teams and have five minutes to think of as many different uses of an elastic band as possible. The team with the largest number of uses wins.

A possible list could include the following:

1   hold papers together
2   attach as a tourniqué
3   attach to a mask
4   use as a spectacle holder
5   use in artwork
6   uses of a giant rubber band include a trampoline, a means of holding timber together, and a launch for a missile
7   use as jewellery
8   hold pencils together
9   sling
10   catapult
11   make musical sounds
12   hold clothes together.

You will find other 'energiser' exercises scattered through the book (e.g. Exercise 17.2 in Chapter 17 on evaluation, and Exercise 23.1 in Chapter 23 on written and audiovisual aids to learning).

Exercise 1.5 Some 'endings'

Most participants will remember very little detail from the learning event as the months progress. As 'endings' tend to be remembered more than other elements of the workshop, they provide an opportunity to reinforce lessons, continue friendships and form networks. They may also provide positive and constructive feedback.

I'm glad I came because ...

To encourage positive feedback and introduce a 'feel-good' factor, each individual is asked to start a sentence with 'I'm really glad I came because ...' and to finish the sentence in whatever way they choose. This continues until there are no more statements to be made. This could be continued with another round, starting with 'I was lucky to be here because ...'. In a similar vein, participants could start a sentence with 'In the future I will do one thing differently, which is ...'. These statements could be collated on a flip chart and action plans developed by considering when and how things will be done differently.

I have appreciated others' company because ...

A list of all of the participants is given to each individual with the instruction to write underneath their name 'I have appreciated this person's company because ...'. This again is a 'feel-good' exercise, and it often gives rise to constructive, positive feedback.

You will find other 'ending' exercises in the book in various chapters (e.g. Exercise 17.1 in Chapter 17 on evaluation).

2

The learning environment: establishing a learning culture

The image of teaching that many people have is that of a teacher transmitting facts while students passively receive this information. Fortunately, this is a fading image as a new generation of teachers offer a new educational environment in which students are more active in their learning.

The educational environment and climate[1-3]

The medical educational environment is complex. Learning takes place in different places and at different times through a variety of methods and activities. The many settings in which learning takes place include lecture theatres, seminar rooms, hospital wards, laboratories, libraries, consulting rooms and occasionally even patients' homes. There are many factors that can influence the environment, including the socialising influences of fellow students, teachers, colleagues, patients, etc., and the sometimes competing aims of the individual, the health service, and the hospital or practice. It is important that the educational environment positively fosters co-operation, supportiveness and learning. The educational climate is the 'personality' attributed to the educational environment. Other terms that have been used to describe the environment's characteristics are its atmosphere, ambience or tone. The climate is very influential on the outcomes of learning, and establishing the educational climate has been rated as the 'single most important task of the medical teacher'.[2]

Box 2.1:

The educational climate should be:
- 'warm'
- supportive
- positive

continued overleaf

- one of trust between participants, where the natural desire to learn can be nourished
- exciting.

It should encourage:

- learner-centred/self-directed learning
- shared decision making
- a journey of emotional discovery
- confidence building.

Learning is optimal when students and their teachers negotiate the purposes and methods of learning in a climate of trust between participants. This partnership between the teacher and the learner should be enabling. The learner must be able to ask questions without fear of being humiliated (this was all too common an experience in medical education in the past – echoes of Sir Lancelot Sprat!).

The teacher needs to be someone who empowers the learner and enables learning, and is therefore more correctly called a facilitator. A key role of the facilitator is to use their educational knowledge and skills to select an appropriate method of teaching and learning for the student. Ideally, the choice would be negotiated with the current learners, but more often choices are made based on discussions with, and feedback from, previous learners.

Planning: think first about the aims and objectives

Whatever teaching method is selected, it is essential that the aims and objectives are clear and based on the needs of the learners. If the objectives are clearly stated, then it is possible to match teaching or learning methods to enable you to plan an activity or programme of learning to achieve those objectives.

The setting of educational objectives should ideally be shared with the learners, taking into account the ability of the learner (or in groups, their differing abilities) and their preferred learning style. The evaluation should be formative and participatory.

JoHari window

The JoHari window[4] is a useful concept for understanding the function of feedback and group and interpersonal activity in the identification of both strengths and learning needs. Figure 2.1 illustrates this concept.

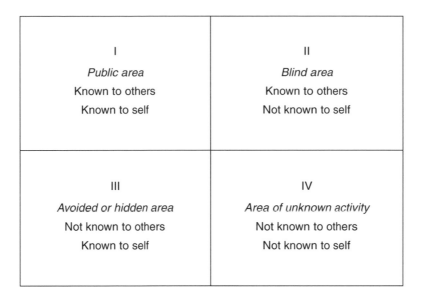

Figure 2.1: JoHari window.

In a new group, or in a new environment, the area in quadrant I is small and that in quadrant III is large (*see* Figure 2.2).

As a group matures, or as people get to know the individual better, quadrant III shrinks and quadrant I enlarges. Poor communication inhibits the enlargement of quadrant I.

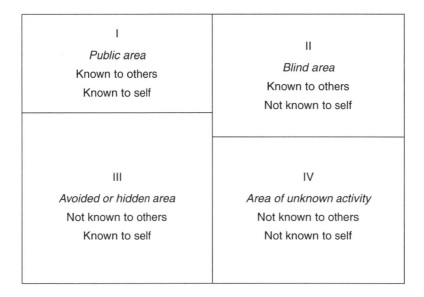

Figure 2.2: JoHari window for new groups.

The quadrants on the right, especially quadrant II, are susceptible to feedback from others, and reducing this area increases the individual's awareness of his or her strengths and learning needs.

Challenge from group members or other external factors reduces quadrant IV and increases the size of quadrants I and II. Internal monitoring also helps to reduce the size of quadrant IV, so that qualities, skills or abilities in this area can be uncovered and moved to quadrants I or III.

There is universal curiosity about quadrants III and IV, but this is held in check by custom, social training and fear of what might be revealed. Teachers and learners need to be sensitive to the covert aspects in quadrants II, III and IV and respect the desire of individuals to keep them hidden.

Note that the JoHari window is named after Jo Luft and Harry Ingham, not Johari!

The application of different teaching methods

It is important to recognise that no single method of teaching is the best one. There are times when the teacher needs to pass on a body of knowledge by selecting a lecture method, and other times when small group work or personal study is more appropriate. What is always important, however, is the quality of the educational climate created by the teacher/facilitator.

The lecture method

This is a good method for transmitting information to a large audience at relatively low cost. Lectures have gone slightly out of fashion in recent years, but they remain an important teaching method in the educator's armoury.

The key to a successful lecture is the preparation and creation of a stimulating educational climate.

Keep the title of the lecture simple and interesting, and remember to introduce the subject and explain the aims and objectives of the session at the beginning! It is well known that people lose their concentration if lectures are unbroken for more than 20 minutes, so why do most lecturers 'bang on' for almost an hour of unbroken speech? The lecturer's aim is not to read to the learner without interaction, but to explain the subject, allowing time for questions. It is wise to plan the lecture in sections punctuated with space for dialogue with the learners, when questions may be asked and points clarified. One way is to pause, perhaps by summarising or using a joke. Another approach is to use an activity break. This might involve asking the learners to turn to their neighbour or to form a small group of three or four colleagues in order to discuss a point or solve a problem (*see* Box 2.2). The break will allow them to think about the issues raised in the preceding section and refocus their attention for the next section. At the end of the lecture it is important to summarise and allow time for the learners to raise any final points and questions.

Box 2.2:

Good examples of activities during a lecture include asking the learners to work on their own or to turn to their neighbour or form a group with three or four others to consider or discuss the following:

- a clinical problem or scenario
- the advantages or disadvantages of a procedure or course of action
- an ethical dilemma
- issues raised in a videotape clip (e.g. of a doctor–patient consultation or a clinical procedure)
- the application of something suggested by the lecturer to their practice
- a statistical question
- an examination question (e.g. a multiple-choice question or an example of a typical viva/oral question)
- the preparation of questions to ask the lecturer
- a cutting from a newspaper (e.g. a patient's complaint, hospital-funding issues, rationing, etc.)
- a reading from a book or a poem related to issues raised in the lecture.

Handouts are often given out at the end of lectures, accompanied by an audible groan as many of the audience will have copied down every word and diagram. Tell the audience if you are going to give them a copy of your slides, but preferably prepare a brief, structured handout allowing space for the addition of notes. Hand it out at the start of the lecture, and allow a few minutes for the audience to scan the paper. One well-received tip is to remember to give the audience any relevant references. This will allow them to concentrate on your presentation rather than trying to copy down text which is often barely readable!

The clarity of the presentation is important. This includes the clarity of the oral presentation and the use of any visual aids. Aids should help to retain the attention of the learner, reinforce the lecturer's main points and actually enhance participants' interest in the subject. Illustrations and diagrams should be colourful and simple. The use of videotape and computer-generated images (e.g. PowerPoint) should enhance the lecture and not distract the learner.

The most important thing to remember is that a good lecture depends on good preparation as well as good presentation!

Small groups

By the term 'small group' we mean a group of from three to about 20 participants. Groups of 5–12 participants are the optimum size. Small groups are
sometimes run as seminars, tutorials and learner sets or team meetings. They
are an increasingly common method of learning, particularly in hospitals,
on wards and units and in the primary care setting of a practice. They
are potentially more intimate and interactive than a large lecture, and are
therefore particularly suitable for interprofessional and team-based learning.

Creating a stimulating educational climate is vital to the effectiveness of a
small group. Careful planning and skilled facilitation are essential. It is important to be in comfortable surroundings that are free from the interruption
of bleeps and telephones.

Small groups work best when all of the participants can see each other
(unlike the backs of heads seen in lecture theatres). Chairs arranged in a circle
encourage discussion and allow both verbal and non-verbal communication
between participants. It is wise to remove tables and other barriers from
within the circle, as the power of non-verbal communication is very important
to the functioning of the small group. The informality and lack of anything to
hide behind helps the group's educational climate to develop.

Ground rules should be explicit and negotiated at the beginning of the
session (*see* Chapter 1). It is important for the participants to feel 'safe'.
The educational climate is further enhanced by encouraging the learners
to prepare for the discussion. Use 'ice-breakers' and other games to facilitate
discussion and allow the members of the group to bond.

The group can also be divided into pairs or trios for more intimate
discussion. At the end of the session it is important for the facilitator to draw
everything to a conclusion, summarise and allow time for the learners to
clarify points of concern. If the group is to meet again, start planning the
following session together.

Ward rounds

The ward round has been and probably still is the centrepiece of a hospital
doctor's learning. Ward rounds have been the occasion of ritual humiliation
of some young doctors, but many others will have had positive learning
experiences on ward rounds over the years. The ward round is a form of
small group activity that usually includes the presence of a patient. Just like

any other small group activity, trust between the participants is necessary. Humour is an important aspect of learning, but it should not be at the expense of the learner or the patient. The good teacher will have agreed the aims of the teaching before the round started, and will have ensured that the educational opportunity that results from the presence of the patient is maximised.

Concentrate on eliciting physical signs and discussing treatment options and differential diagnoses whilst communicating with the patient. A good teaching ward round should be planned, with the learning objectives defined for each of the patients concerned. This is followed by a discussion after the round that will enable the learner to discuss different aspects of the cases in the privacy of a room away from the patients.

One-to-one learning

The tutorial is the formal setting for one-to-one learning, but valuable learning can also take place informally in the workplace, at the bedside, in the consulting room, etc. Again the learning environment and the climate generated are all-important. The learning will be more effective if the room is comfortable and free from interruptions. Time must be protected. The aims and objectives need to be planned and based on the needs of the learner as for any other learning activity. Feedback to the learner must be positive and constructive, and it is also important that both the learner and the teacher evaluate the session.

Tutorials are ideal opportunities to indulge in role play or to watch video-tapes of the learner's (or teacher's) consultations in a safe environment. Similarly, in-depth discussion of a specific patient's problems using random case analysis and critical-event analysis are ideal approaches for the intimate environment of a one-to-one tutorial.

Tutorials are best when they are planned, but *carpe diem* encapsulates the concept that learning opportunities can be fleeting moments that should be grasped firmly as they arise. This may be following a ward round, in the ward office or in the common room after a general practice surgery, or in the car between domiciliary visits. Look out for opportunities, and seize the day!

It is important to remember the effect that the teacher has on the tutorial. Just as the learner will have a preferred learning style, the teacher will also have a preferred teaching style which could have a powerful effect on the dynamics of the one-to-one learning experience (as, of course, does the learning style of the learner).

Quirk[5] describes four types of teaching styles:

* *assertive*: extrovert and tends to direct the process by leading from the front
* *suggestive*: tends to offer ideas and thoughts readily

- *collaborative*: identifies and legitimises the learner's difficulties
- *facilitative*: encourages the learner to discover the way forward by using and developing their own skills.

This model should not be interpreted as meaning that the facilitative style is the one that should always be used. An under-confident learner may need the teacher to give an answer, or may need prompting. Teachers should understand the effects that their preferred style could have on one-to-one learning, and adapt to the situation as necessary.

Many factors may impair the one-to-one educational experience (*see* Box 2.3). Both teachers and learners should be aware that the quality of the learning experience depends on both of the participants. Time should be spent at the end of the session reflecting and discussing how the process could be improved even further (remember to be positive) and planning for the next time.

Videotaping the tutorial and watching it at a later date with the learner can help to improve the skills of the teacher and highlight the behaviours of the learner, provide an opportunity to pick up on specific points, or be a trigger for further learning opportunities.

Box 2.3: Factors that impair one-to-one learning[1]

Learner	*Teacher*	*Learner/teacher*
Poor preparation	Too technical	Poor rapport
Poor confidence	Too didactic	Collusive
Anxiety	Too talkative	Allow parent/child relationship to develop
Introversion	Too impressive	
	Too self-centred	
	Too judgemental	
	Too attentive	

References

1 Middleton P and Field S (2000) *The Trainer's Handbook*. Radcliffe Medical Press, Oxford.

2 Genn JM and Harden RM (1986) What is medical education here really like? Suggestions for action research studies of climates of medical education environments. *Med Teacher.* **8**: 111–24.

3 Chambers R and Wall D (2000) *Teaching Made Easy*. Radcliffe Medical Press, Oxford.

4 Luft J (1970) *Group Processes: an introduction to group dynamics* (2e). National Press Books, Palo Alto, CA.

5   Quirk M (1994) *How to Learn and Teach in Medical School.* Charles C Thomas, London.

Games, activities and learning techniques

Exercise 2.1   How we learn

Why you should do this

You hope that the participants will see that workshops help with learning.

When to use this

When people are learning about learning, or are new to learning. It is useful when people have raised doubts about active learning and expressed a wish to be passive and listen to 'talks'.

What to do

Ask participants to write down on a piece of paper something that they are good at. Then ask them to write a few words on a 'post-it' note about how they became good at that activity. Collect the 'post-it' slips and stick them (lightly) on to a flip chart. Read them out, and then ask the group members to suggest some general headings under which to clarify the various activities and methods of improvement that they have recorded.

How it works (insight)

It provides participants with an exercise in which they can all take part whatever their previous experience. You can modify your approach to the learning styles of the participants. The group members can see that they learn best from experiential learning, and feel more positive about active learning.

Whom to engage

This exercise can be used with anyone and everyone.

How much time you should allow

Allow the participants one minute for thinking of something they are good at, and three minutes for recording how they became good at it. Allow about 10 minutes for discussion and drawing out the common themes.

What the facilitator should do

Move the exercise along quickly. Do not suggest the ideas that participants might record when giving the briefing.

What to do next

Draw attention to the classifications. They will always include the following:

- learning by doing
- practice
- learning by mistakes
- some flippant remarks.

There will be little reference to 'being taught by sitting and listening to someone'.

Another idea for developing or adapting this exercise is to repeat it but this time focus on what people are 'bad at' rather than what they are 'good at'.

What makes it work better

A good variety of participants from different backgrounds and with interests outside their work.

What can go wrong

Some people may take the exercise too light-heartedly and write down ridiculous things that they are good at, or provide frivolous examples of how they became expert in these activities.

3

Running small groups

Small groups are a good format for encouraging participants to interact, explore and develop ideas and challenge preconceived beliefs. Small group work promotes critical and logical thinking as part of a problem-solving approach. It is a useful approach when building up a team to help group members to understand why other members hold different views and what 'makes them tick'.

The task for the group should be wide enough to encourage participants to own and develop the topic themselves, but also focused enough to restrict the ensuing discussions to the matter in hand.

With sufficient time, a small group will evolve through five stages of development in group dynamics:[1]

1 *forming*: getting to know one another
2 *norming*: working out the norms, roles and goals of the group through informal discussion. There may be expressions of uncertainty about the task and some frustration about lack of progress
3 *storming*: leaders emerge and some group members are perceived by the others as having special talents. The group may become emotionally charged, with some members becoming angry or impatient
4 *performing*: decisions are reached, and tasks are sorted out with mutual support and individual satisfaction. The group ends by reviewing and summarising its achievements
5 *mourning*: the group begins to disband as time runs out and members reluctantly leave the group.

Tips for organising small group work

- Limit the numbers in a small group to twelve, but preferably six or eight.
- Arrange the chairs in a quiet spot facing each other in a circle so that all members feel equally part of the group and can easily see everyone else.
- Remove any empty chairs so that the group feels complete.
- Appoint a small group leader or a facilitator who is skilled at handling group dynamics.

- Start the small group work by welcoming everybody in order to create a positive atmosphere in the group. Introduce yourself and ask the others to do the same.
- Agree the ground rules for the group, including confidentiality, listening respectfully to each others' views and comments, deciding whether mobile phones should be switched off, punctuality, regular attendance, etc.
- Make sure that everyone knows what the task is, and reinforce this with a written description of the task.
- Brief the facilitator or group leader well before the session, so that he or she knows what main points should emerge from the discussions, and can guide the group members back to the central task if they become side-tracked.
- Invite someone other than the facilitator to monitor the timing of the task(s), to encourage group ownership.
- Encourage someone other than the facilitator to report the group's discussion back at a subsequent plenary session. Choose this person at the beginning of the group work so that they can prepare to report.
- The facilitator should reflect any questions back to the group, so that rather than being seen as acting as an expert, they draw others in to respond instead.
- Ensure that everyone has a chance to contribute by indicating to dominant members that they should talk less, and encouraging quiet members to participate.
- Keep to time, and pace the group work appropriately to complete the task.
- Draw the group to a final ending. The facilitator could summarise the main points, provide positive feedback, look at future development needs, or invite participants to give positive feedback about the event or their interaction with other group members.

Problems with groups and group members

Box 3.1:

What can go wrong with the way in which a small group functions

- The small group may be ill-balanced, with some members forming an excluding clique that stifles discussion and exchange of ideas.
- Inadequate introductions mean that no one knows who anyone else is or what their backgrounds are.

continued opposite

- Group rules of conduct about confidentiality or the boundaries of discussion are not aired or agreed, so that participants feel inhibited about divulging sensitive information. Even worse, group members do confide sensitive information which is relayed outside the group later on.
- Too many small groups packed into the confines of one room mean that group members have difficulty hearing what others are saying, and are distracted by what the other groups are doing.
- Too little time is allowed for the small group work to address the set task.
- One or two members dominate the group whilst others sit quietly and are not engaged.
- At the report-back session the group member presents his or her own views instead of the essence of the group's discussions.
- Participants may have hostile, preconceived views about the small group approach. They may feel that their time is being wasted by learning from each other rather than listening to an 'expert', or they may chat instead of addressing the task.

Dysfunctional groups include the following categories.

1 *Cliques that have beliefs which seem strange or unrealistic to outsiders.* The group regards as disloyal, or imposes sanctions on, any group member who deviates from these beliefs. The group often regards itself as superior to outsiders and is resistant to change. Some trade unions behave like this – and many religious organisations do, too! Working groups in organisations may develop such behaviour.

2 *Dictatorships that are based on the cult of obedience to a strong leader.* Many general practices seem to have been (or perhaps still are) run like this. Occasionally the dictatorship can be seen as benign – for example, the individual may be exceptionally talented – but as is shown elsewhere in this book, teamworking produces better results than individuals working alone.

3 *A group that lacks a clear function.* This has the following characteristics:
   - some members making irrelevant and excessively long contributions
   - the same points coming up at every meeting
   - discussion tending to focus on abstract issues or generalisations about how people are feeling, rather than on concrete practical matters or reports of evidence
   - some members regularly failing to attend, or making no contribution to the meeting
   - decisions never seeming to be made, and everything always going forward for further consideration

- decisions being made outside the group that make group discussions irrelevant.

Such groups are often set up 'to be seen to be consulting the staff' or 'to build team spirit', but all meaningful communication and decisions are made elsewhere. The solution is to determine the purpose of the group (e.g. if the purpose is to obtain feedback about decisions made elsewhere, then a mechanism to show that the feedback is effective is required). If the group has no real function apart from a social one, then the group members are better off going to a social meeting place, such as the pub.

4 *Powerless groups that lack economic force, control of information or authority.* For example, the group may come to the conclusion that a particular action is required, but have no authority or access to funds to make it happen. The solution is to include these resources in the group structure.

Dysfunctional groups may involve the following difficult dynamics and processes.

1 *Pairing*: two group members may talk quietly to each other rather than participating in the group discussion. This is distracting and irritating both to the group and to the facilitator. Sometimes the pair will always discuss things across the group with each other, rather than involving the whole group. This can also occur when there is another 'expert' or 'star' in the group with whom the facilitator prefers to interact because they are 'on the same wavelength'. You can:
   - suggest that the group members change seats to perform certain activities, or after reconvening
   - ignore the problem (it sometimes resolves if the members begin to interact with the rest of the group)
   - ask the two group members to share what they are discussing with the rest of the group
   - draw attention to the problem and ask the group how they would like it to be resolved.

2 *Scapegoating*: where one or more of the group members frequently attack another member. You might:
   - suggest taking a short break, or switch the discussion (this may only provide temporary relief)
   - draw the group's attention to the process and suggest that it may be a defensive manoeuvre for the whole group with regard to their feelings of aggression that need to be expressed more openly
   - use humour to point it out each time it happens to enable the participants to stop the behaviour.

3 *Projecting*: where one or more of the group members identify their own feelings as apparently coming from the group (e.g. 'this group is very

angry'), when in fact only one or two members are showing that emotion.
The whole group may project emotion, becoming caught up in circular
discussion about 'the dreadful management' or 'the incompetent government'. You might:

- offer the idea of a group projection to the group and see what they
  make of it
- ask the group to identify what is happening (this approach is best for
  an experienced group)
- ignore the problem and move on to another topic.

4 *Subversive subgroup*: where a dominant person draws into discussion
   adjacent group members, who form a hostile and sarcastic group, challenging the facilitator and the work of the group. This needs swift action,
   such as the following:

- the facilitator expresses his or her disquiet at what is happening, and
  asks the group how the activity can be modified to meet the aims of all
  members of the group
- the rest of the group is asked what is happening (but they may feel
  powerless or reluctant to confront the hostility)
- direct confrontation, although this can backfire unless the facilitator
  can isolate the ringleader, and it may lead to a battle.

5 *Wrecking*: this is a one-person variant of the above and tends to be more
   overtly confrontational. The individual may constantly disagree with or
   refuse to take part in activities. He or she may arrive late, walk out of the
   group, or express displeasure by facial grimaces, sighing or restlessness.
   The wrecker will often have been 'sent' to the group. You might:

- talk to the person on their own outside the group and try to reach an
  understanding of their behaviour
- draw the group's attention to the person's behaviour and ask them to
  suggest the reasons for it
- confrontation occasionally works if the behaviour has not been too
  overtly hostile and has been unconscious – but it can also be met by
  denial and a power struggle.

6 *Flight*: one or more group members may change the subject, make a joke
   or become silent. This often signals that the emotional intensity in the
   group has become too great, sometimes because of personal identification with the subject matter (*see* Chapter 6). You might:

- ignore it if it does not interfere with the work
- point it out as a group process and see what happens
- encourage it (as you encourage the group to change tack or laugh,
  they will recognise why they needed to do it and learn to tolerate the
  emotion)
- guide the group back to the difficult area (this approach is necessary
  when emotional issues are the focus of the group activity).

7   *Shutting down*: this occurs in an individual as a more extreme reaction
     to a situation that causes flight – it is an 'internal flight'. It occurs in
     situations where emotions are engaged or a hidden agenda is suddenly
     revealed. You might:
     •   allow the person 'time out' to recover
     •   show understanding by means of a touch or look
     •   change the subject
     •   take the person aside after the group meeting and ask if he or she
          would like help or support outside the group to deal with the issues
          that have been revealed.

8   *Rescuing*: this is the opposite of scapegoating, where one or more group
     members constantly act to protect another member. Sometimes the person
     who is being rescued sets him- or herself up by playing 'poor me' games.
     The process can paralyse a group and prevent both the rescuers and the
     rescued person from acting as adult learners. Try:
     •   asking the rescued person what they want to do
     •   consulting the group about what is happening and what should happen
     •   confronting the rescuers
     •   drawing parallels between what is happening in the group and the
          subject under discussion, if this is relevant.

9   *Hidden agendas*: work agendas include anxiety about how the individual's
     performance is perceived by others from the same work environment,
     especially if managers are present. Interpersonal agendas include people's
     own concerns about themselves (e.g. worrying about whether the leader
     likes them, or whether the group members think they are stupid or too
     talkative). Other hidden agendas can include covert hostilities that have
     developed between group members, or difficulties that have been brought
     in from other environments, such as disagreements at work or in a social
     context. For example, two doctors from a partnership that has split up are
     going to find it difficult to work together in a group where they have to
     co-operate! You might:
     •   use the ground rules exercise (*see* Exercise 6.1)
     •   use the feedback rules (*see* Chapter 1)
     •   invite the group to explore what is happening
     •   ignore the problem if it is not interfering with the learning activity too
          much.

     You can often modify the behaviour of difficult individuals by asking
     them to perform specific tasks. For example, you might ask them to help
     the facilitator to arrange the room or collect papers, or ask them to work
     with another group member (who is either more experienced and sensible,
     or in need of support, as appropriate).

Some of the material from this section is derived from Chambers R and
Wall D (2000) *Teaching Made Easy.* Radcliffe Medical Press, Oxford.

Reference

1   Walton HJ (1973) *Small Group Methods in Medical Teaching.* Medical Education, Book 1. Association for the Study of Medical Education, Dundee.

Games, activities and learning techniques

Exercise 3.1 Working in trios

Why you should do this

Learning as a trio encourages interactivity. If a problem is presented from real life, this immediately engages the participants, as it is building on their experience and is relevant to their situation – the criteria of successful learning described in Chapter 1.

When to use this

To encourage a wider perspective on any situation that the participants may encounter in their everyday work (e.g. for problem solving or learning consultation skills).

What to do

Three people make up each small group (a trio) who sit together where they can talk and listen to each other in a quiet place. A task involving role play might be set by describing a problem-centred scenario that is relevant to the topic being taught. Alternatively, each member of the trio might present a relevant problem issue for them, employing the problem-solving technique. Use the letters A, B and C to designate the members of each trio group. Their roles are as follows:

* role of A: to present an organisational, social, personal or professional problem to B
* role of B: to examine and define A's problem
* role of C: to observe the interaction between A and B, and to keep time.

A and B talk and interact whilst the exercise progresses through the following sequence:

1   problem presented
2   problem examined
3   problem defined
4   solution proposed

5   solution discussed
6   solution implemented
7   review exercise: self-assessment by B, feedback by C to B, and feedback by
     A to B.

C acts as timekeeper, stopping the role play or alternative exercise at the pre-agreed
time, and monitoring the length of the debriefing period. If there is time, repeat
the exercise twice with each member of the trio taking turns at being A, B and
C, presenting a problem, examining it and observing the others' interaction.

   If the number of participants is not a multiple of three, arrange for one or
two groups to have four members, with two people taking the observer's role
each time.

How it works

Each of the three participants sees the problem from three perspectives – that
of the person with the problem, that of the person who is trying to solve the
problem, and that of the observer looking on. All of the participants realise
the others' perspectives for themselves – a powerful mode of learning. If a real
problem is posed, the trio will usually generate more options for solutions
than a single participant working alone would have done.

Whom to engage

Any three peers.

How much time you should allow

The time allowed will depend on the problem or topic being presented, and
how long it takes to describe a problem and discuss a solution. The role play
should take at least ten minutes, with a further ten minutes for debriefing,
giving a minimum of 20 minutes in total for each role-play episode.

What the facilitator should do

Explain the task clearly, as learners often have difficulty in understanding
exactly what is required of the A, B and C roles. Keep an eye on the pre-agreed
timekeeping for each stage, and remind C if the exercise is running over time
or being foreshortened. Remind the participants to give positive feedback
rather than dwelling on what might have been improved.

What to do next

Encourage the participants to decide on their own action plans, building on
what they have learned from the exercise.

What makes it work better

- A theme for the trio work that is relevant to all of the learners.
- Sometimes A, B and C are termed the 'explorer', 'guide' and 'observer', respectively. These terms describe the roles that they play in presenting a real problem to explore, and in guiding the 'explorer' towards identifying his or her options for solutions. The guide could ask the explorer what he or she would like to have achieved to be able to judge the trio task as a success – to establish the boundaries for the discussion. The guide should find out whether the explorer has reached the limits of their understanding of the situation and, if so, extend their horizons.
- The facilitator could draw up a summary sheet for the observer to use to record their notes (*see* the example below).

What can go wrong

- Participants who are 'senior' in real life may not act as 'peers' to the others, so that those who are playing the A, B and C roles feel constrained with regard to the interchange of the trio work and in giving feedback.
- The participants become so engrossed in a real-life problem that they lose touch with the reality of the exercise and divulge sensitive information or become emotional.
- The participants do not grasp the task, and C interrupts the interchange between A and B rather than quietly observing.

Example of a summary sheet that an observer (C) might complete in an exercise where the trio work concerned a patient (A) with a psychosexual problem in consultation with a doctor/nurse (B)

Agree on the number of minutes to be allocated to discovering what hidden problem the patient has, and then discuss this for the agreed time.

Observer's tasks

- Keep the 'doctor/nurse and patient consultation' to the agreed time limits.
- Write down your comments on the consultation.

After the agreed time stop the 'consultation' and:

- ask the 'doctor/nurse' to state what he or she thought the hidden problem was (i.e. self-assessment)

- ask the 'patient' to state what the hidden problem was and what the barriers to telling the 'doctor/nurse' were
- ask the observer to comment on the interactions that they noticed
- have a discussion about how the problem might be managed differently
- summarise the action points in the table below.

Points observed during the 'consultation' (prompts to consider are listed below)

- Were leading questions used?
- Were the questions closed or open?
- Were non-verbal clues picked up?
- Was there a flexible or rigid approach?
- Was the vocabulary suitable for the patient or too clinical?
- Was the doctor/nurse making assumptions?
- Was the consultation focused on the problem?
- Was time well used?

Points observed:

Use the prompts below during the discussion.

Which questions or phrases would have helped a shift to include a psycho-sexual history from this patient? Write some exact wording.

continued opposite

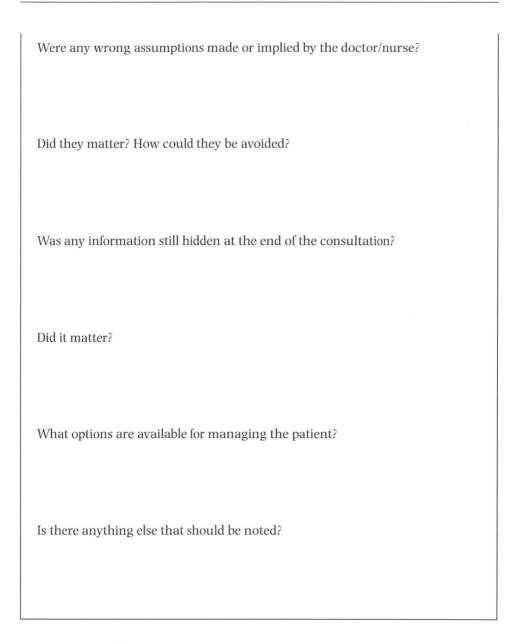

Were any wrong assumptions made or implied by the doctor/nurse?

Did they matter? How could they be avoided?

Was any information still hidden at the end of the consultation?

Did it matter?

What options are available for managing the patient?

Is there anything else that should be noted?

Exercise 3.2 Goldfish-bowl technique

Why you should use this

It will help participants to become aware of other people's perspectives on a situation, and it will encourage reflection on performance, communication skills, alternative approaches to difficult problems, and lateral thinking in problem solving.

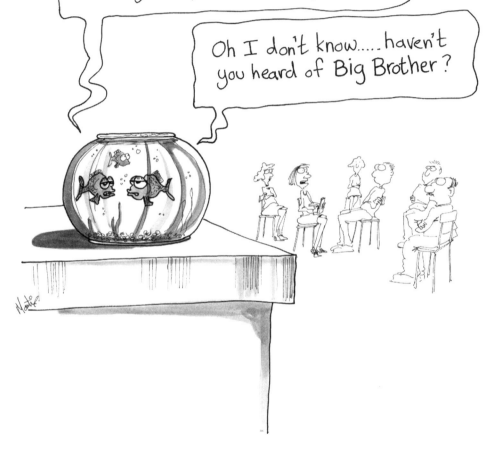

When to use this

You could use this technique in a workshop setting where group rules have been established and people who are part of the 'inner' group feel safe when undertaking their task whilst being watched by those in the 'outer' group.

What to do

1 Position the seating in a private room so that people sitting on chairs in an 'outer' ring can observe the two or three people who are sitting together in an 'inner' group. Members of the inner group sit facing each other with their backs to the outer ring of participants.
2 The people in the inner group perform a task, such as undertaking a role play set by the facilitator. For example, they might act out a scenario in which a senior person counsels a junior individual about his or her performance.
3 First the inner group may feed back their observations and feelings as to how the task went, followed by the outer group giving feedback of their observations. Alternatively, the 'inner' and 'outer' group discussions may be held separately, after which the two groups come together so that everyone can hear what the others think. Feedback should be positive and supportive (*see* Chapter 1).
4 Finally, the whole group discusses the task, performance, observations and learning points facilitated by the teacher.

How it works (insight)

The organisation of this exercise encourages observation and reflection. It is often difficult to see your own mistakes because you are too close to the issues involved. The 'goldfish-bowl technique' allows participants not only to stand back and observe a situation relevant to their own experience being played out, but also to exchange ideas with others about what could be done better, and to share good practice.

Whom to engage

This exercise allows people who do not like undertaking role play to observe from the outer circle, as only a few participants will be required in the 'inner group'. The technique is suitable for any discipline or level of seniority. Two facilitators might act out planned good practice or planned bad practice in the centre of the 'goldfish bowl' to start the exercise off.

How much time you should allow

The time taken will depend on the nature of the role-play exercise. Allow a minimum of 10 minutes for the role play, followed by at least 20 minutes for the inner group and outer circle discussions, and additional time for drawing out the overall learning points.

What the facilitator should do

Explain the arrangements for the exercise clearly so that those in the outer group understand that they must keep quiet and observe whilst the role play is in progress. Set out the task for those doing the role play so that they cover all of the ground necessary to bring out the key learning points that match the objectives of the exercise. Insist that the 'rules' for giving positive feedback are adhered to, and encourage wide-ranging discussion.

What to do next

Consider running a second exercise using the goldfish-bowl technique with a revised role play and task that have been informed by the discussion of the first round.

Encourage individual participants to devise an action plan based on what they have learned from participating in the role play or observing it, and to record their learning in their personal portfolios.

What makes it work better

- Ask for volunteers for the role play, rather than press-ganging reluctant individuals into taking part.
- Choose a role play and task that are immediately relevant to everyone's situation and learning needs.

What can go wrong

- Participants in the outer group may ignore the rules about giving constructive feedback in a positive manner, and launch into negative comments about the performance of those in the inner group.
- Too little time may be allowed for discussion and extracting the overall learning points of the exercise.

4

Communicating better

Why we should improve our skills

We all think that we know about communication skills, and are often baffled when someone misinterprets something that we have said or done. Yet on another level we are just as aware of all the pitfalls – for example, the time when we made a joke and the recipient took offence, or when we received a message that made our blood boil or which was totally incomprehensible.

No one should be so complacent that they feel they cannot improve their communication skills. You can categorise people into one of three levels as follows.[1]

1 *Unskilled*: People at this level use whatever methods come naturally, good or bad. They have little or no insight into the effect that their communication has on other people, and they tend to blame others for failures or dismiss others as hopeless or incapable of changing. Rude bullies in the workplace often feel that they are doing well. What they do not realise is that their subordinates avoid them and conceal much of the day-to-day business from them. They become isolated and out of touch with what is actually going on (most dictators eventually fail because of this).

2 *Using acquired tricks*: At this level people have learned some useful communication skills, but they tend to apply them uncritically without observing their effect and the feedback from others. We have all encountered people who listen intensely to whatever is said and respond inappropriately with expressions of great sympathy, or offer coping strategies, when all the speaker was doing was providing a superficial social interchange. Others sigh, look pathetic or drop hints, rather than simply stating what it is that they want.

3 *Skilful communicators*: people at this level have a wide range of appropriate behaviours that can be tailored to the situation and modified according to the feedback that is received. It may sometimes be appropriate to give didactic orders (e.g. to shout 'fire – everyone out') or to drop gentle hints when someone is sensitive ('perhaps you would like to confine the minutes of this meeting to just the summary points?').

Improving communication skills

You can learn how to observe, evaluate and change the way in which you communicate with other people. Receiving feedback from others will help you to make the necessary changes. Other areas that can help include the following:

- techniques (e.g. presentation skills)
- flexibility (e.g. it is useful to have a loud voice and project it to the back of the room if one is speaking in a hall with no microphone, but not appropriate to use it when talking one to one or in a small group)
- knowledge (e.g. of the signs that indicate a person's background mental state) (*see* Figure 4.1) can help you to understand not just what is being said, but also the feelings behind the words.

The meaning of language

Most of the time we understand what people say, but sometimes our 'wires get crossed'.[2] Some examples of poor language skills are listed below.

- *Taking things literally*. The answer to the question 'Have you seen that file I put down?' is not 'Yes', but 'It's over there on the table'.
- *Action meanings*. People often use action statements when they do not like to ask directly for things. Saying 'It's very fresh in here with the window open' can be a request for the window to be closed, and the speaker will be quite offended if you reply 'Yes, it's nice to have some fresh air'.
- *Connotative meanings*. These can suggest emotions but express what is said and what is meant differently. Many people remember their full name being used when someone was telling them off. People who use metaphors which imply that the workplace is a war zone (e.g. we shall attack this problem on several fronts and defend our position on this matter) may be expressing their inner feelings about it being a battlefield. A reply that is entirely appropriate in a social setting may be regarded as offensive in a work environment (e.g. after someone has spent hours preparing a document, the response should be a proper appreciative message, not a scribbled note saying 'thanks, OK').
- *Using jargon*. The use of jargon can sometimes be an unconscious attempt to prevent communication and understanding. After all, if you do not understand what I am talking about, you cannot possibly do my job! More often it involves failure to use the feedback (or lack of it) to modify what is being said to suit the level of understanding of the listener.
- *Using formal or informal styles in the wrong settings*. People speak in a different way to their friends to that in which they converse with colleagues or

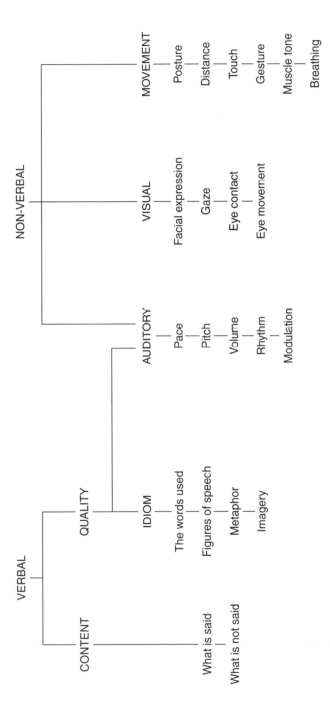

Note: bear in mind that cultural factors may influence what is happening (e.g. the amount of eye contact, gesture or touch may be altered according to the culture of origin or adoption).

Figure 4.1:   Signs of the mental state in communication.

people at work with whom they have an unequal power relationship. You may encounter someone using a 'chat-up' style with a colleague, or introducing their partner as Mr or Mrs Smith at an informal get-together in a pub. Generally, the more formal the event, the more formal the language, and some people find it difficult to gauge the right level. Cultural factors affect the situation – what might seem excessively formal to an American may seem over-casual to someone from Japan.

References

1   Reid M and Hammersely R (2000) *Communicating Successfully in Groups*. Routledge, London.

2   Hargie ODW (1997) *The Handbook of Communication Skills* (2e). Routledge, London.

Games, activities and learning techniques

Exercise 4.1   Ice-breakers and rounds

Why you should do this

Ice-breakers are an introduction to communicating with verbal and non-verbal language. You can use rounds to provide a quick interchange of personal information that enables the group members to start their communication (*see* Chapter 1 for more details about ice-breakers).

When to use this

You might use ice-breakers and rounds:

* at the start of a workshop
* at the beginning of a new session
* to begin a new topic or phase
* to end a topic or phase.

What to do

The minimum activity is just to have a round of names, but you can add to this by including some information from each participant. It is often helpful for the facilitator to write down the information on a flip chart or white board so that people can continue to refer to it. Drawing a circle and putting in the names helps both the leader and the group to recall who is who. Comment on how the words that people use can sometimes mean the same thing, although they are phrased quite differently, or that similar wording can have different connotations. If this exercise is done at the end of a session, you might comment on any obvious differences between individuals in the ways in which the same communications in the workshop have been heard and assimilated.

1 *Introductions*: set the style by introducing yourself and mentioning by what name you would like to be known, and ask each person to do the same.
2 *Introductions and information*: make the criteria explicit by asking each person to give their name and one or two sentences about one of the following:
    - why they have come to the workshop
    - what work they do
    - one memorable fact about themselves – give examples such as 'I used to have green dyed hair' or 'I really like visiting art galleries'.
3 *Starting a topic*: you might like to establish a baseline by asking people to give one or two sentences about the following:
    - any previous experience they have of this topic
    - what they would like to gain or learn from this session
    - what this topic means to them.
4 *Setting the agenda*: ask each person to write down on a 'post-it' note up to three things (one per post-it note) that they would like to achieve during the workshop. Stick the notes on a flip chart and classify them with the help of the group. Then ask the group to try to put the items in order of priority and add any others that seem to be as important.
5 *Finishing off before a new topic or phase*: you can use a round to summarise before moving on. Ask people to write on a post-it note one thing that they will remember or have learned from this session, or one thing that they intend to do as a result of the session. Put these comments on a flip chart and share them with the group by trying to classify them as a summary to the session.

Other ice-breakers were described in Exercise 1.3.

How it works (insight)

The interchange of names and some information helps to move people towards feeling more comfortable with each other (i.e. moving from storming and norming to forming a group) (*see* Chapter 3). Communication is increased as people feel more free to speak once others have revealed a little of themselves to the group.

Whom to engage

Any group that is starting up or moving to a different topic, or a group that starts to fragment into subgroups and needs to be pulled together. Rounds are useful when returning to the large group from twos or trios.

How much time you should allow

For introductions and information, allow only about two or three minutes per person. Starting or finishing a topic might need a little longer (three or four minutes) per person. Setting the agenda needs about four or five minutes for writing down ideas, 10 to 15 minutes for writing them up and classifying them, and about 10 minutes for arranging them in priority.

What the facilitator should do

Make the atmosphere calm and welcoming so that people feel comfortable. Set out the rules clearly and keep to time. Encourage the quiet members to participate, and subdue the noisy ones with verbal and non-verbal signals.

What to do next

Move on to other more specific exercises to look at, for example, language confusion.

What makes it work better

*   A small group of people who are used to working in groups with a variety of different participants.
*   Articulate participants with audible voices, and a quiet enough room for everyone to hear them.
*   Asking for volunteers to start if the group is a new one, and selecting people who have not had a chance to speak if it has been going on for some time.

What can go wrong

*   The group may be too large. If there are more than 16 to 18 people, rounds become tedious and people (including the facilitator) cannot remember who said what.
*   If the group is dominated by someone who hogs the limelight or talks for too long, people will become embarrassed or bored.
*   If the group contains people who do not want to contribute, the others may feel too exposed to criticism by those who are not similarly vulnerable.

Exercise 4.2 Fly on the wall

Why you should do this

It illustrates the difficulty of obtaining a complete picture of an action or intention without being able to test out your conclusions.

When to use this

The participants need to have some pre-planned action that has not yet been discussed in the group. You might have asked each participant to bring an idea that they would like to see implemented, which others in the group would not know about. You could use action plans discussed in pairs or in another group composed of different members. You could supply a selection of ideas from a range of objectives – you will need one per participant in the small group, or less if time is limited. For example:

- how to move some sheep from an island that will be flooded when the river rises another metre
- how to protect an electricity substation from a lava flow from a volcano
- how to move an elderly person from a house that is going to be knocked down to build a motorway
- how to organise a rescue for someone who is stranded on a rock in the sea in a foreign country
- how to prevent people from tipping rubbish in a beauty spot.

What to do

Divide the larger group into smaller groups of four or five people. Ask for one person from each group to choose and 'own' an objective as if it were their own project, which is written as the heading on a flip chart. Give the owner of the first objective a pad of paper and a pencil.

The rest of the group will discuss how to fulfil the objective. The owner must remain completely silent – a 'fly on the wall' – and privately record notes on what is proposed.

Each owner takes it in turn to remain silent and record the discussion until the time is up (there will probably only be time for two or three objectives to be discussed in each group).

Then the owner of each objective presents what he or she thought the action plan should be, *and* what the group had proposed as far as he or she had understood it, by writing up a summary under the heading on the flip chart. After the presentation, the other group members point out any discrepancies between what they thought they had agreed and what the observer had concluded. The observer should write these discrepancies in a different colour on the flip chart. The whole group can then draw conclusions.

How it works (insight)

It draws attention to how difficult it is to be certain what action others intend to take when you cannot check with them in order to remove any misconceptions. Your idea as the owner of an objective may be different to that of a group set up to implement it.

Whom to engage

This exercise is particularly useful for groups who are having to set objectives and make action plans in their workplaces.

How much time you should allow

Allow 5 to 10 minutes to set up the groups and for each participant to choose an objective. (You will need about 10 to 15 minutes if the participants bring their own objectives to write on the flip chart.)

Allow 15 minutes for discussion of each objective, so two objectives in each small group will take about 30 minutes. In the large group, each presentation should be written up in about 8–10 minutes, and discussion following each presentation allowed for about 5–10 minutes. (Discussing six objectives takes about 1½ to 2 hours in the large group.)

What the facilitator should do

Prepare some objectives, even if you have asked the participants to bring them (almost certainly several people will forget). Keep a close watch on the 'flies on the wall', encouraging them just to record and not to speak. Help the large group to pick out discrepancies between the observer's conclusions and the small group's decisions. You could summarise any general learning points about communication skills and difficulties.

What to do next

Ask the participants for their thoughts about how they can improve communication when drawing up and implementing action plans.

What makes it work better

- Using objectives that are not familiar to the small group discussing them.
- Using examples that are not drawn from the work situation ensures that the observer does not make correct assumptions on the basis of previous experience, but has to depend on the group communication.
- Groups of four to five people work best – that is, enough to generate discussion and different ideas.

What can go wrong

- The 'fly on the wall' may find it impossible to remain silent and may join in the discussion, or try to put people right about what is intended.
- One member of the small group may take a dominant role and dictate a clear course of action.
- The small group may be too large and may thus lose sight of the objective.

Exercise 4.3   Where are you from?

Why you should do this

To facilitate the group's cohesion and provide examples of communication.

When to use this

At the beginning of a group, or when reforming a group after a significant break, to augment previously acquired information and remind everyone about the identity of the group members.

What to do

Have a large map of the world, the country, the county or the city that can be spread out on the floor. Participants are asked to go and stand on the following areas in turn:

- where they were born
- where they live
- where they work
- where they did their training.

Each time, ask them to state who they are, where they are, and a short sentence about why they are there.

How it works (insight)

It reinforces the learning of names, and enables some self-disclosure that makes the group more comfortable later when disclosing other matters such as feelings or opinions.

Whom to engage

New groups with members who are not known to each other.

How much time you should allow

Move quickly from one statement to another, only allowing a few minutes for each participant to exchange a couple of sentences each time. The whole exercise takes about 30 minutes.

What the facilitator should do

Move people quickly, and stop (tactfully) anyone who gives a long explanation of where they are (e.g. 'Hey – I'm sure that's three sentences so far!'). Move past anyone who is looking really uncomfortable, and allow them not to move if necessary.

What to do next

Move on to the next activity.

What makes it work better

Participants who are unknown to each other and who have moved around the county or country a lot.

What can go wrong

- Most people come from one area, and the one or two who come from other areas feel excluded (check the participants' addresses before you use this ice-breaker).
- For some people there may be parts of their life that they do not want to reveal.

5

Examining attitudes

Why should we need to examine attitudes?

Our internal values modify our behaviour, by allowing or forbidding certain actions. Judgements about what needs to be done are often made not because of our skill or training, or because of logical analysis of the evidence available, but because we think 'it is the right thing to do' or 'it is in the best interests of the person or organisation'.

Decisions about what we do need to be constantly re-examined against the general ethical and moral order. This is complicated by the fact that we live in a multiracial, multicultural society. Attitudes that are acceptable in one sector of society may not be generally applicable in other sectors. Standards that were regarded as acceptable a few years ago may be seen as dangerously dogmatic now, as ethical and moral judgements are modified (e.g. the issue of consent for organ removal after death).

If we are to learn to be as non-judgemental as possible, we need to recognise and acknowledge our attitudes towards other people's life situations, beliefs and feelings of independence. Just as we may be unaware of our learning needs (the unconscious incompetence in JoHari's window; see Chapter 2), we are also unaware of our prejudices unless we take deliberate steps to identify them.

The codes of conduct for nurses and doctors require them to respect the beliefs of patients and not to impose their own attitudes on them. There are many examples of cases where this is simply not being followed. For example, homophobic attitudes have been recorded in many research papers.[1,2] The feelings of loss of control, vulnerability and isolation that accompany illness leave many people vulnerable to manipulative behaviour by their carers and health workers.

Negative attitudes and expectations prevent good services from being accessible to all. Embarrassment, negative previous experiences and concerns about confidentiality and lack of respect create barriers between people and the services that they need. Lack of appreciation of different language or language usage, cultural differences and social exclusion increase these barriers.

Autonomy and paternalism

In the past, the relationship between patients and health staff, or between solicitors and clients, relied heavily on paternalism. An imbalance of power was created by the superior knowledge of the provider of services. A failure to communicate was explained by the attitude that the patient or client would not understand the complex decisions that had to be made. This stance is untenable in an era of increasing dissemination and availability of information. This autocracy is challenged by the patient or client who attends with an Internet printout of more information than the doctor or solicitor knew existed.

We need to consider how to move from autocracy to the following.

- *Partnership*: help for someone with a problem comes through partnership between that person and the professionals.
- *Empowerment*: the professional's role is to help to empower those with problems to find the best ways of helping themselves.
- *Judgement*: beware of judgement – the person with the problem is the only one who really understands their experience and problems.
- *Values*: people's values and priorities change with time, and they may be quite different from your current values, but no less valid.
- *Autonomy*: this should be a fundamental right of every individual. Illness, disability, low income, unemployment and other forms of social exclusion mean a loss of some aspects of autonomy in society.
- *Listening*: this is the most important word for any professional. Active non-judgemental listening is the core art of helping people, and is crucial if one is to gain an understanding of people with problems.
- *Shared decision making*: people with ongoing problems need to be able to take their own decisions about the management of their clinical condition, based on the expert information that is communicated to them by professionals. Shared decision making leads to concordance.
- *Concordance*: a negotiated agreement on the management of a clinical problem between the person with the problem and the professional[3] allows the patient to take informed decisions on the degree of risk or suffering that they wish to take on. In contrast, 'compliance' with treatment, lifestyle or other changes implies that the patient or client follows instructions from professionals to a greater or lesser degree.

Meaningful involvement of the public[4] and needs assessment

The resources allocated to the health and social services or to education or housing, etc., are related to the importance attached to those services by the political party in power in government. Managers and workers in those sectors have a duty to provide the best services possible within the constraints of the available budgets. The assessment of needs by the managers, or by the people providing the services, may not coincide with that of the wider public, or with the needs of an individual. The conflict between the duty to provide the best service possible and the budgetary constraints may provide impossible ethical dilemmas. Concordance, discussed and negotiated between individuals or groups of people, can provide answers. However, many professionals have attitudes that lead them to persist in trying to provide services when resources are clearly inadequate, or deciding to suspend them, rather than establishing priorities with the people for whom the services exist.

References

1   Naji SA, Russell IT, Foy C *et al.* (1989) HIV infection and Scottish general practice: knowledge and attitudes. *J R Coll Gen Pract.* **39**: 284–8.

2   Faugier J and Wright S (1990) Homophobia, stigma and AIDS – an issue for all healthcare workers. *Nurse Pract.* **3**: 27–8.

3   Royal Pharmaceutical Society of Great Britain (1997) *From Compliance to Concordance: towards shared goals in medicine taking.* Royal Pharmaceutical Society of Great Britain, London.

4   Chambers R (2000) *Involving Patients and the Public: how to do it better.* Radcliffe Medical Press, Oxford.

Games, activities and learning techniques

Exercise 5.1 The human bar chart

Why you should do this

This exercise enables participants to express their attitudes without being able to modify them by checking how others are receiving them. People cannot go along with the majority. Some attitudes will be exposed as requiring examination and thought.

When to use this

You might use this exercise before any activity that will require people to be as non-judgemental as possible. Taking a sexual history, learning counselling skills, and teaching about parenting or relationships are all areas where it has been found to be useful.

What to do

The facilitator writes out a list of statements that might represent people's attitudes, as in the list given below. Reproduce each statement on a separate sheet of flip-chart paper. Hang each up along one wall of a room, allowing enough space for people to stand in lines in front of each statement.

Examples of statements that could be used include the following.

A   Homosexual acts are unnatural.
B   If a girl under 16 years of age asks for contraception, her parents should be told.
C   Abortion should be available on demand.
D   Condoms should be available in secondary schools.
E   Sex outside marriage is wrong.
F   The age of consent for gay men should be raised back up to 21 years.
G   The subject of gay and lesbian issues should be taught in schools.
H   Homosexuals are more promiscuous than heterosexuals.
I   Sex is unnatural in the over-50s.
J   Girls should be expected to control the sexual behaviour of boys.

Give each participant a piece of paper listing the statements with a marking grid (*see* opposite). Make sure that there is enough room between each line to fold over the paper to obscure the answer. Read out each statement and ask the participants to circle their attitude towards the statement quickly on the marking grid. Each person marks *one* statement and folds over the paper. The group member passes the marking grid on to the next person, and each marks the next statement, folds over the paper and passes it on.

When all have been completed, each participant folds the entire grid in half and then passes it across the group at least three times. Everyone should have a marking grid by the end of this process.

Ask the participants to unfold the marking grid. Read out the first statement again and ask people to stand in a line *according to the grade given by the marking grid*. Repeat the process for each statement, recording the number of people in each grade for each statement. When you have finished, the participants return to their seats and the facilitator leads a discussion about the results.

Marking grid:

Circle the number which represents your views or feelings about each statement

STRONGLY AGREE   to   STRONGLY DISAGREE
A   1----------------2----------------3----------------4----------------5----------------6

STRONGLY AGREE   to   STRONGLY DISAGREE
B   1----------------2----------------3----------------4----------------5----------------6

STRONGLY AGREE   to   STRONGLY DISAGREE
C   1----------------2----------------3----------------4----------------5----------------6

STRONGLY AGREE   to   STRONGLY DISAGREE
D   1----------------2----------------3----------------4----------------5----------------6

STRONGLY AGREE   to   STRONGLY DISAGREE
E   1----------------2----------------3----------------4----------------5----------------6

STRONGLY AGREE   to   STRONGLY DISAGREE
F   1----------------2----------------3----------------4----------------5----------------6

STRONGLY AGREE   to   STRONGLY DISAGREE
G   1----------------2----------------3----------------4----------------5----------------6

STRONGLY AGREE   to   STRONGLY DISAGREE
H   1----------------2----------------3----------------4----------------5----------------6

STRONGLY AGREE   to   STRONGLY DISAGREE
I   1----------------2----------------3----------------4----------------5----------------6

STRONGLY AGREE   to   STRONGLY DISAGREE
J   1----------------2----------------3----------------4----------------5----------------6

How it works (insight)

People express their attitudes privately without consultation. They are often surprised to find the extent to which other people's opinions differ, having assumed that everyone thought the way they did.

Whom to engage

Anyone and everyone.

How much time you should allow

Nine statements will each take one or two minutes to mark and exchange the grids. Forming the human lines will take up to 30 minutes (more if there are a lot of people). The discussion should be fairly brief, lasting about 20 to 30 minutes.

What the facilitator should do

Make sure that everyone understands that the marking on the grid is private and should be respected. Stop anyone unfolding the paper to look at a previous answer. Move the pace for the marking on the grid along briskly so that people do not compare answers or have time to think which answer is 'the right one'. Keep the discussion at the end brief, moving on from one statement to the next quite quickly, especially if anyone looks uncomfortable.

What to do next

Move on to looking at ways of examining participants' own prejudices and making changes, or move on to the main task for which this is a preparation.

What makes it work better

- A group of about 15 to 30 people is best. It is possible to do this exercise with really large groups (e.g. a lecture theatre full) by using a show of hands rather than lines of people and recording the numbers on a chart.
- You could modify the exercise for use with an electronic voting machine.
- It has more individual impact in small groups.
- It works best if participants are prepared to be honest about their responses.

What can go wrong

- Participants may take too long over their responses and try to guess what answer is expected.

- Participants may compare answers (this is common in large groups where supervision is a problem).
- People may be so embarrassed by the realisation that they were in a minority that they are either unable to contribute to the discussion or else put up defences against the rest of the group.
- Participants may make disparaging remarks about other people's attitudes either in the lines or in the discussion.

Exercise 5.2 The lifeboat and the island

Why you should do this

This exercise helps participants to look at and discuss their attitudes to people.

When to use this

Before planning changes to services.

What to do

Make a collage of the photographs of a number of people cut out of magazines or newspapers. Using velcro pads, stick them on to a picture of a large boat. Choose 'typical' examples to represent the various categories of the population. You might choose 10 to 12 different types from people recognisable as:

- elderly
- physically handicapped (e.g. in a wheelchair)
- mentally handicapped (e.g. with Down's syndrome)
- blind or wearing thick spectacles
- deaf, with a hearing-aid
- homosexual
- black
- Asian
- a strong man
- a weak man
- a woman in her twenties
- a woman in her forties
- a child
- a baby
- a famous singer
- a nurse in uniform
- a soldier in uniform, etc.

Tell the group that these people are in a lifeboat travelling towards an unin-
habited wooded island. The lifeboat will only reach the island if a maximum
of six people are in the lifeboat. Divide the participants into small groups of
four to six people and ask them to decide who will stay and who will leave,
giving the reasons behind the decisions. Then reconvene in the large group
and consider each character in turn. Stick each one to a flip chart divided into
two columns, headed 'for' and 'against'. Encourage discussion of the judgements that are made.

How it works (insight)

This exercise reveals much about how we judge others and their 'worth'
to society. It can help people to realise that many of their judgements are
superficial and hasty.

Whom to engage

Groups who are going on to draw up plans for services or setting priorities or
categories for treatment within a budget.

How much time you should allow

Explaining the task and dividing into groups takes about 5 minutes. Allow
40 to 45 minutes for discussion in the small groups, and about the same
amount of time for the feedback and discussion in the large group.

What the facilitator should do

Prepare the characters to be easily recognisable, and have a few spare ones
available. Prevent the discussion from becoming personalised. For example, if
there is someone in the group who would fit a particular character, substitute
another. Divide the groups so that they are well mixed. Keep to time, and
encourage discussion and a light-hearted approach.

What to do next

Move on to the main task.

What makes it work better

- A mixed group of people from varied backgrounds and disciplines.
- Avoiding personalised statements.

- Encouraging a light-hearted approach and emphasising that this is a game.

What can go wrong

Taking it too seriously, identifying with one of the characters and making personalised statements (e.g. 'That's my granny you're throwing overboard').

6

Understanding feelings

Why do we need to recognise feelings?

Many of us learn to hide, ignore or minimise our feelings. We try to believe that we are rational and logical, and that feeling upset or showing emotion – especially in the work situation – helps no one, least of all ourselves. On the contrary, recognising and understanding the emotions generated in ourselves and in others helps us to understand better what is going on and how to manage the situation. By not using our emotional reactions we are wasting a valuable resource.

Feelings unconnected to the immediate situation

You or someone else may have an emotional reaction due to something outside the current situation. For example, perhaps you are in a meeting and someone looks distracted and answers angrily when asked for their opinion. You later find out that they had a car accident on the way to the meeting.

Indirectly connected emotions

Sometimes called 'resonance', this occurs when a situation or person reminds you of another about which you have experienced considerable emotion. For example, you explain to a receptionist that you have an appointment with someone in the building. You feel very angry when the receptionist tells you to sit down and wait to be fetched, and you recognise that her attitude and speech remind you of a teacher who always made you feel small and inadequate. Sometimes this 'resonance' can provoke some-one into behaving inappropriately – perhaps shouting at the receptionist or refusing to wait.

Directly connected feelings

You may respond directly to something that another person presents, either consciously (e.g. by bursting into tears), or unconsciously (e.g. with aggressiveness of speech or posture).

Dealing with the feelings

Most of the time what we feel is a mixture of all three of the above categories. We take our prior emotions with us into any encounter, perhaps a sense of calm or happiness if things have been going well, or haste and confusion if they have not. We may recognise the echo of our previously experienced emotion in an inappropriate reaction to something or someone – or we may be baffled by the way in which we responded. We may need to reflect sensitively to someone else how the emotion in the room is making us feel – for example, 'It seems to me that you have some strong feelings about what has happened?'.

Sometimes we just try to ignore the emotion, especially if it is one that we have brought into the situation from outside. If it is minor, we may succeed in this approach, but if it is overwhelming, everyone else will be aware of it and the sufferer will miss much of what is going on in an effort to control their feelings. If your emotional state is likely to affect your relationship with others, it is wise to mention the cause and to apologise for your distraction. If you do not, others may take your response personally and assume that it is connected with them in some way.

'Acting out the feelings' is an approach that parents often adopt. Looking stern, sounding concerned or allowing a little anger to show can sometimes be helpful. Perhaps if someone is feeling guilty or ashamed, showing a little condemnation may relieve the other person from bearing the emotion alone – as long as they do not feel rejected. Using phrases such as 'I expect you are feeling really bad (or angry with yourself) about that' shares the emotional response without rejection. Occasionally allowing someone to see that they have driven you beyond a controlled response can make them see that changes have to be made – again so long as they are not totally overwhelmed by your response. However, if you find yourself constantly losing control of your feelings, you would be better off deciding to deal with them in some other way, or taking avoiding action.

Using the feelings that are picked up from someone else in a constructive way can be really useful, and can often move people towards making changes. This approach is frequently used in the interactions between patients and health professionals. For example, you might observe that a female patient always becomes very defensive when talking about her husband. This may provoke the response that the patient's mother always criticises him, so his wife feels that she has to stand up for him – but she feels he is actually too weak to do this for himself and she despises him for it. In a meeting, you might notice that the chairman always defers to the man who sits opposite. During a break, you might comment to the chairman on this man's air of condescension and boredom. The chairman might look thoughtful and seek to avoid looking at that person in the latter part of the meeting, perhaps recalling previous similar scenarios.

Difficult feelings

People who sexualise what would otherwise be a work-related interaction cause great difficulties. Sometimes it is possible to draw their attention to the nature of the interaction and point out that it is inappropriate. Sometimes they are unaware that this is how they always behave. For example, children who have been sexually abused may react in this way, leaning against you and stroking your arm or leg. At other times you may feel so alarmed that your only recourse is to arrange for someone else to deal with them, after explaining to the other person what the problem is, in fairness to them.

Feeling depressed can also present problems. You may not realise how you are colluding with someone until you catch yourself agreeing that 'nothing can be done'. By its very nature, depression reduces communication and puts up barriers against action and resolution, and can be a useful clue when the presentation of a problem does not fit any recognisable pattern. Anxiety may be just as inhibiting, especially to health professionals or managers who prefer to operate in an environment of certainty. The anxiety may be that of the health professional or manager – being unsure how to proceed, or concerned that something is seriously wrong. On the other hand, the anxious feeling may be coming from the patient or staff member who is concerned about your reaction, or about what is going to happen.

Although good feelings can often be accepted as your just reward for a job well done, beware the person who makes you feel special by telling you that you are the only one who can help or understand them. You may be manipulated into restricting your actions in order to keep pleasing this person, and if you find that this happens often, you may need to examine your own motives for 'needing to be needed' in this special way.[1,2]

References

1   Freeling P and Harris CM (1984) *The Doctor–Patient Relationship*. Churchill Livingstone, Edinburgh.
2   Berne E (1996) *Games People Play*. Ballantine, New York.

Games, activities and learning techniques
Exercise 6.1 Setting ground rules

Why you should do this

Agreeing ground rules is a way of making a contract of behaviour at the start of a workshop, and can be used to explore feelings about previous learning experiences (*see* Chapter 1 for more details).

When to use this

At the start of a new group.

What to do

This exercise is easier with two facilitators. One can record while the other draws out the contributions from the group. The facilitators should feel free to contribute – it is their group, too! Draw three columns on the flip chart or board, one headed 'rule', the next headed 'why' and the third headed 'feelings'.

Explain the need for 'ground rules' or a 'group contract'. Invite the participants to suggest rules, and ask them to explain the reasoning behind their suggestions. You will find that most of the rules suggested are due to negative or favourable previous experiences. Ask the participants to state what they felt about what happened previously, as well as giving an account of what happened. Encourage discussion by asking how other group members would have felt in the same circumstances.

How it works (insight)

People will be less likely to be disappointed or frustrated by the behaviour of others. This exercise increases understanding of the behaviours that they prefer, and of those behaviours that prevent learning, and how both of these affect other people.

Whom to engage

This exercise is useful for the beginning of any group, particularly when the participants are not known to each other, or if there have been any signs of behaviours that are counter-productive to learning as the group assembles.

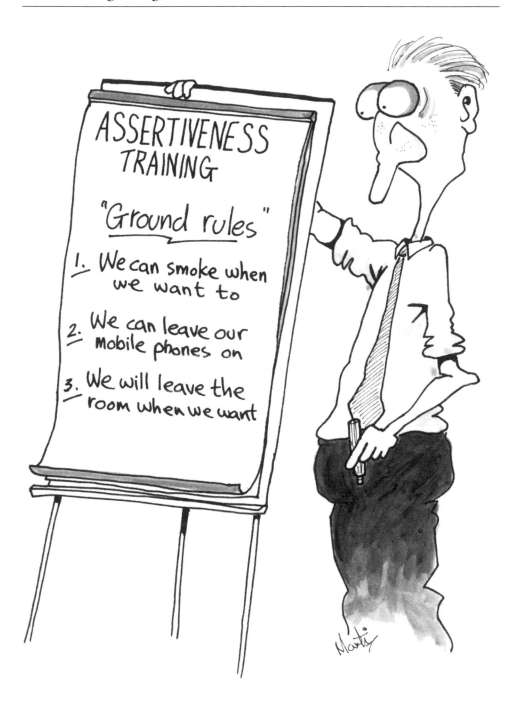

How much time you should allow

You will need enough time to explore each suggestion. Allow at least 45 minutes (more if it is a large group).

What the facilitator should do

Try to ensure that everyone has an opportunity to contribute. Add any suggestions that you consider the group has omitted. Be prepared to explain why and what feelings that behaviour produces.

What to do next

Proceed with the rest of the workshop.

What makes it work better

Participants who have previous experience of group work and reflective practice.

What can go wrong

- Participants may not take the task seriously and may propose facetious rules.
- The facilitator may lose control of the group before the ground rules can be set, and is thus undermined.
- Many group members may arrive late and so feel excluded and not bound by the rules that have been set by the others.

Exercise 6.2 Bringing out the feelings

Why you should do this

To establish that it is acceptable to talk about feelings, and to look at ways in which feelings can be discussed.

When to use this

During the reflection at the end of a section or at the end of a workshop, particularly if the participants will be meeting again.

What to do

The facilitator introduces the subjects by writing up headings on a whiteboard or flip chart. Record the feedback from the large group under the following headings:

- perceptions
- feelings
- thoughts
- behaviour.

Under *perceptions*, ask the participants to describe their own and other people's actions during the previous section of the workshop. Ask them to list what were the best and worst things about that section.

Then under *feelings* ask them to describe the following:

- how they felt during that section
- what other feelings this produced
- how they feel about this now.

Under *thoughts*, ask them to describe the following:

- what the things they have observed mean
- what they can learn from them
- whether there were any surprises
- the significance of the findings.

Under *behaviour*, ask the following questions and record the answers.

- What are you going to do as a result of your conclusions so far?
- How can you apply what you have learned?
- What are the risks of acting on your insights?
- How can you use the insights to your advantage?
- What other options would you have in a similar session?
- Will you do anything differently as a result of the session?

You may find that people are moving between the various headings, in which case allow them to go with the flow rather than sticking rigidly to the divisions. Having all the headings visible at one time makes it simpler for the facilitator to record the feedback.

How it works (insight)

Discussing the feelings produced by the work and the behaviour in the group reduces the uncertainty in the group about the underlying reasons for the responses of the participants about the learning.

Whom to engage

This exercise is particularly useful for groups that will continue to work together over a number of workshops, or for a team that is taking forward an action plan.

How much time you should allow

The exercise takes about 30 minutes for a small group of six to seven people, and twice as long for a larger group of 12 to 14 people, to allow everyone to describe how they felt and the insights gained.

What the facilitator should do

Record the insights, clarifying with the participant if necessary, but without putting your own interpretation forward. The insights should be those of the group participants alone. Only make suggestions if the group members do not understand the nature of the task. Encourage everyone to participate, and do not allow any one person to dominate the proceedings with his or her own perceptions to the exclusion of others.

What to do next

Start a new section of the workshop or prepare for the next one, asking the participants to take away the insights they have gained to use on the next occasion.

What makes it work better

- Describing what went on in small groups in the plenary group usually goes well, as people are naturally curious about what others were doing.
- Having two facilitators means that one can prompt the group while the other records.
- It works best with a lively interactive group who do not mind expressing their feelings.

What can go wrong

- People may not want to reveal how they feel because they have inappropriate feelings, or their feelings are making them uncomfortable.
- People may be unskilled in how to express their feelings without blaming others for how they have responded.

- The facilitators may be too hurt by adverse criticism to respond profes-sionally, and they may become defensive.

Exercise 6.3   Reverse rounds

Why you should do this

This exercise allows participants to express how they are feeling and to acknowledge that it is useful to do so.

When to use this

If the session is flagging, or if there are hidden currents preventing work.

What to do

Ask the participants to turn their chairs outwards so that they are facing away from each other. The facilitator then asks the group members to shut their eyes and think, or preferably write down for themselves, how they want to complete a sentence. Ask people to use the sentences to feed back how they actually feel – if they can. You can use all or some of the following suggestions.

- What I like about this workshop is ...
- What I find difficult in this workshop is ...
- I find it useful to work in this group because I feel ...
- What I would like more of in this group is ...
- What I would like less of in this group is ...
- What I would like to do next is ...

How it works (insight)

Saying how one feels without being able to see other people's responses helps to free participants to be more honest.

Whom to engage

Any group that is stuck, or for a light-hearted interlude after a serious or frustrating subject.

How much time you should allow

Allow only about half a minute's thinking time to complete each sentence, before going round asking people to read out their own completed ones.

What the facilitator should do

It is important that the facilitator moves people on quickly, and allows individuals to refrain from contributing if they feel that they cannot do so.

What to do next

Take up the suggestions that have been made if they are practical, or explain why you cannot if not.

What makes it work better

- A group that is prepared to be honest in their replies.
- A group of 8 to 12 people.
- A facilitator who is prepared for criticism and can handle a joker.

What can go wrong

- Too small a group (less than four people) makes any criticism of the group seem too personal.
- Too large a group (more than about 12 people) makes the activity tedious.
- Having one or more jokers who make facetious remarks all the time can be disruptive and inhibitory to others.

7

Teamwork

All groups of people are composed of different types of individuals with differing needs and agendas. The behaviours that are present and the atmosphere which they cause all contribute to the group dynamics – the interrelationships that occur when groups of individuals work together.

If the group or team is dysfunctional, conflicts arise and relationships come under pressure. Resentment and general discontent may develop, leading to factions in the team and the taking of sides, which often results in the eventual breakup of the group or team.

Teams may break down as a result of poor management, lack of guidance, poor communication and lack of support. Games are often instigated by people who want to hang on to power, and who may feel insecure or threatened by others. Power is something that people will try to grab, steal or manipulate. When power in any organisation is abused or mismanaged, the results will inevitably lead to a dysfunctional work environment.[1]

If managers are equivocal about teambuilding, and the staff members that attend teambuilding activities are the least influential ones who can most easily be spared, the long-term result will be that nothing will change. Failed attempts to improve team relationships will simply reinforce the staff's cynicism.

Teambuilding starts from the top. When power is well managed, it can encourage security, support and trust, with frank and open discussion and negotiation – all components of teambuilding. Without this, no organisation will be able to function to its full potential. Teambuilding takes time, effort and consistency, but is rewarding.[1]

Effective teams make the most of the different contributions of individuals. Your team is more likely to function well if:

- it has clear team goals and objectives
- it has clear lines of accountability and authority
- it has diverse skills and personalities
- it has specific individual roles for members
- it shares tasks based on individuals' strengths, weaknesses and interests
- it regularly communicates within the team, both formally and informally
- it has full participation by team members
- it confronts conflict

- it monitors team objectives
- it gives feedback to individuals
- it gives feedback on team performance
- it has external recognition of the team
- it has two-way external communication between the team and the outside world
- it offers rewards for the team
- it provides opportunities for self-development.[2]

A team leader with a democratic style enables a team to function well and encourages, rather than imposes, change.

Good communication in teams

Good communication is essential for good teamwork. You need:

- regular staff meetings, which managers and staff endeavour to attend
- a failsafe system for passing on important messages
- a way to share news so that everyone is promptly notified of changes
- a culture in which team members can speak openly without fear of being judged or reprimanded
- opportunities for quieter members of the team to contribute
- to give and receive feedback on whether your role in the team is succeeding in its objectives
- to praise others for their achievements
- opportunities for team members to point out problems and suggest improvements
- everyone to be part of and to own the decision making.

Communication is usually poor if a team lacks stability, or if single disciplines work in an isolated way. In one study,[3] some of the senior doctors were the worst offenders in terms of failing to communicate with others in the team. Power and status issues within a team can interfere with good communication.

References

1   Chambers R and Davies M (1999) *What Stress in Primary Care!* Royal College of General Practitioners, London.

2   Hart E and Fletcher J (1999) Learning how to change: a selective analysis of literature and experience of how teams learn and organisations change. *J Interprof Care.* **13**: 53–63.

3   Miller C, Ross N and Freeman M (1999) *Shared Learning and Clinical Teamwork: new directions in education and multiprofessional practice.* The English National Board for Nursing, Midwifery and Health Visiting, University of Brighton, Sussex.

Games, activities and learning techniques

Exercise 7.1 Spot the deliberate mistakes

Why you should use this

To demonstrate that individuals bring with them different skills which, when added together, give a more capable team.

When to use this

You could use this exercise in a workshop on which the topic of the exercise is based to:

*   liven up the meeting
*   encourage collaboration.

What to do

You can reproduce the cartoon (*see* page 75) on sheets of paper for everyone to mark the deliberate mistakes (hazards in our example), and then compare the results as a group. Alternatively, you could reproduce the cartoon as an overhead transparency and the group could identify the deliberate mistakes either as individuals or in pairs, listing their answers on their own answer-sheets.

How it works (insight)

Different people will spot different mistakes that you have depicted. Bring everyone together and pool their observations, and the team should realise that their collaboration has identified many more of the hazards that exist, if not all of them.

Whom to engage

A subject such as 'health and safety', as in our example, should be appropriate when disparate members of a team of varying seniority are attending, as it represents a topic for which they are mainly at the same level. This exercise can be used for:

- any group of individuals – people who know each other, who work together or who have never met before
- people of any level of seniority
- a multidisciplinary mix of learners.

How much time you should allow

Up to 10 minutes for individuals to work alone circling the deliberate mistakes (e.g. the hazards in this example) on the picture, although the exact time will depend on the nature of the mistakes and how obvious they are. You should allow 20 to 60 minutes for the pooling of ideas about the deliberate mistakes, especially if they are likely to be contentious and will trigger the group to discuss what is 'right' and what is 'wrong'.

What the facilitator should do

Stay in the background and let the event happen, be the timekeeper and encourage the group members to pool their views. Intervene if quiet members of the group are not able to contribute to the discussion. Encourage a consensus if the exercise is not coming naturally to a conclusion.

What to do next

Encourage individuals to realise for themselves the value of collaboration. Ask them to identify what factors in the exercise encouraged collaboration (e.g. good skill mix, mutual respect for each other). Encourage them to write an action plan on how to replicate the teambuilding 'in real life'.

What makes it work better

- A topic and cartoon that are relevant to participants.
- Organise participants so that some work initially as individuals and others as pairs. They can then observe the extent to which a 'pair' observes more mistakes than individuals working on their own. The pairs can later combine to form a team.
- Sufficient time to debrief after the exercise and action plan.
- Humour in the cartoon.
- Including deliberate mistakes of which many learners will be unaware, so that there is subsequent discussion and team learning.

What can go wrong

- Because it is a cartoon, the participants may regard the exercise as trivial and fail to extract the learning points and generalise to their 'real-life' situations.
- No one in the group may be aware that some of the deliberate mistakes are 'wrong', and thus opportunities for peer learning are reduced.

Example: spot the hazards of health and safety in an office environment

Look at the illustration below, which shows a rather disorganised workplace that is full of hazards. Try to spot the hazards – they might be found in any office workplace. Many of these hazards might cause back pain from tripping, lifting loads, carrying unwieldy objects, adopting a poor posture, etc. Turn over the page to find the answers.

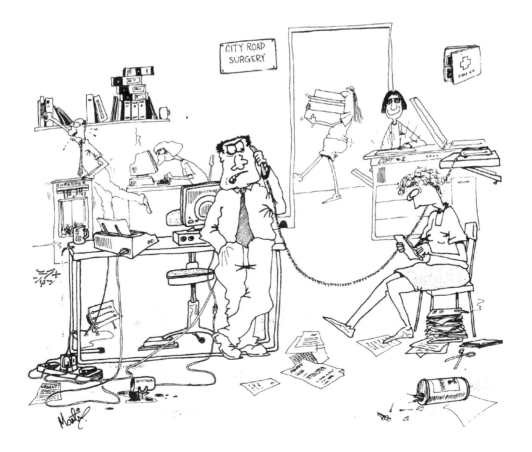

Answers to example

Did you spot the hazards in the fictitious premises? We have found thirty:

1   sharps box on floor spilling out needles
2   coffee cup spilling its contents on to the floor
3   coffee mug by printer has been repaired, so is dangerous
4   trailing wires from the phone, computer and printer
5   overloaded adapter with many wires plugged into the socket
6   open electric fire without guard
7   electric fire is near to trailing lead
8   unattended cigarette butt burning on table
9   secretary's cigarette lying on top of pile of papers by her chair
10 scissors lying open on floor
11 electric lead to computer frayed in the middle
12 computer chair propped up on books because a wheel is missing
13 printer almost falling off edge of table
14 urgent notice lying on floor
15 private letter lying on floor
16 secretary sitting just below telephone shelf, so likely to hit her head when she stands up
17 poor posture of secretary
18 poor posture of computer operator in background
19 dangerous pile of files on shelf
20 coffee mug poised on high shelf above computer operator – hot contents might tip over her
21 man over-reaching for books on high shelf
22 man in background poorly balanced and in danger of catching fingers and tie in the shredder
23 shredder has spilt waste paper on the floor – fire hazard
24 letters on floor by secretary – fire hazard
25 papers and letters on floor create potential hazard which might trip up passers-by
26 woman in background carrying awkward and heavy load
27 photocopier lid open, causing possible eye strain hazard to operator
28 first-aid box has open door
29 mouse hole – there may be vermin
30 overcrowded room – threatens privacy of confidential phone calls.

If you did not spot most of these hazards, get started on learning more about health and safety now!

Exercise 7.2 Write a person specification for an ideal team member

Why you should use this

To provide an opportunity for participants to talk openly about how team members should behave without personalising comments about current team members.

When to use this

When the team is malfunctioning and members want to improve the situation.

What to do

Take a few employee specifications that have already been drawn up for interviewing for various posts – if they exist already. Then select suitable components with regard to the characteristics of the person (e.g. conscientious, good communicator, punctual, etc.). The group can then brainstorm what other components they want to add that describe a good team player. If there are no pre-existing job specifications, the facilitator should draft two or three, as those who have not previously been involved in the interviewing process may not know what an employee specification is. The group should then decide which of the components are 'essential' and which are 'desirable'.

How it works (insight)

This exercise forces the participants to agree on the characteristics of a good team member, and to describe them.

Whom to engage

A current team of people from a workplace, or a newly forming team from several workplaces in order to establish 'ground rules'.

How much time you should allow

There will be considerable discussion of the particular components of the employee specification checklists and whether they are essential, desirable or so unimportant that they can be omitted. Allow up to an hour depending on the number of examples you include.

What the facilitator should do

Find or write a few job specifications as examples.

What to do next

Participants might compare themselves and colleagues against the employee specification checklists and identify gaps in their professional development needs and skills.

What makes it work better

A warm and trusting atmosphere and obvious commitment from the management to take action to improve the team dynamics and expertise as a result of the exercise.

What can go wrong

The adult approach to improvement is wrecked by childish behaviour, barbed jokes and accusations.

Exercise 7.3   A chess set can aid your understanding of relationships and interactions in a quality improvement exercise

Why you should use this

To actively engage a team of people in a 'hands-on' exercise that will help them to understand the different dimensions of a problem, where a move means that the dynamics change as in real life, and where all of the participants can join in.

When to use this

With a small team to encourage collaboration and understanding of team members' roles and responsibilities with regard to those within the workplace and others who work in different health settings.

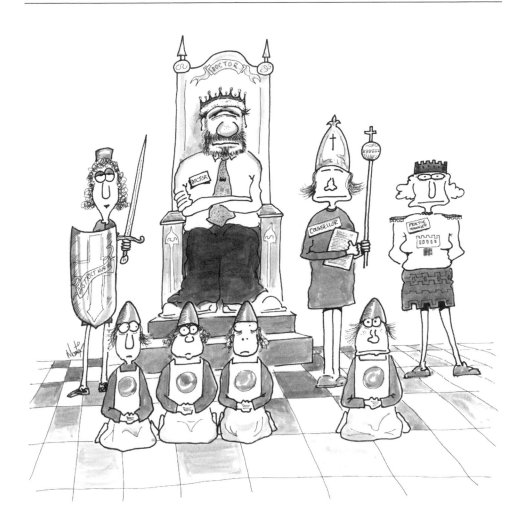

What to do

Sit in small groups of three or four people. Each group has a chess set, a chessboard, a set of chequers and a pad of small (e.g. 2 × 3 cm) 'post-it' notes. Tell the participants that:

- white pieces represent the workplace team
- black pieces represent the patients, clients or customers
- chequers can be used to represent any people who work outside the workplace
- 'post-it' notes can be used to label any piece.

Task 1. Ask the question 'Who will be included in your quality improvement programme in the next 12 months?' Select which of the chess pieces representing your team will be involved. Describe them by name or post on a 'post-it' note and attach it to the relevant chess piece. Arrange your pieces to show how they will work together on the chessboard (e.g. one group or sub-groups). Allow 15 minutes for this task.

Task 2. Ask the question 'What two priority areas will you choose to look at first, and why?'

Review the people and posts represented by the chess pieces. Do you want to change or extend the range and identities of the people you have involved in Task 1?

Rearrange your pieces. Allow up to 30 minutes for this task.

Task 3. Say to the participants 'The government has decided that XXXX is a priority for your patients/clients/customers. How will you accommodate the requirement to improve the quality of XXXX service in your quality improvement programme? Reallocate and rearrange your chess pieces'. Allow up to 20 minutes for this task.

Task 4. Ask the question 'What other resources, people or other thing(s) do you need to take your quality improvement programme forward?' Allow up to 30 minutes for this task.

How it works (insight)

The difficulties of accommodating top-down instructions to practitioners working in a health setting are well represented. The 'hands-on' arrangement of this game engages the players, and the changing situation forces the participants to focus on the roles and responsibilities in the team and to consider how to be flexible in order to accommodate new requirements with the same resources.

Whom to engage

This exercise can be done with a small team who usually work together, or with people from different workplaces so that they can learn how to behave as a team.

How much time you should allow

This exercise takes at least an hour, because of the extent of discussion needed to set priorities, agree changes, etc. The time suggested in the 'What to do' section above adds up to 95 minutes.

What the facilitator should do

Construct a lifelike problem with a scenario setting out local issues and the context. Encourage the participants to think more widely than just their workplace team as they start to deal with more priorities from outside the workplace. Try to emulate multi-agency or multi-sector working in real life.

Emphasise that the activity is not a game of chess, but that it is simply utilising the chess pieces, chequers and chessboard for the purposes of inter-active learning.

What to do next

Make an action plan for teamwork with others who share responsibility for the health and well-being of the participants' patients, but who work outside the health setting.

What makes it work better

Recognisable problems and priority setting with which the participants can identify.

What can go wrong

Participants who cannot play chess may mistakenly believe that they are at a disadvantage.

8

Motivation

Motivation may be positive or negative. It is 'that within the individual, rather than without, which incites him or her to action'.[1]

With *positive motivation*, the individual may be stimulated to learn more or to act differently because of an inspiring teacher, because the subject interests them a great deal, or because they see the great relevance to their future career progress.

With *negative motivation*, the individual may learn or act because of a fear of failure or punishment or threat of other adverse events. The threat of punishment can be a powerful motivating force for change.

Positive motivation leads to deeper understanding and better long-term learning than negative methods, which lead to superficial learning that is often soon forgotten. Motivation seems to be a basic human function. We seek to achieve things, to accept challenges and to work at learning new ideas and new skills throughout our lives. In this area we may assume four principles of motivation.

- We all have a built-in urge to attempt to achieve things.
- Our needs are related to specific goals – factors such as self-image, group bonding and security all have a place.
- The relationship between needs and goals is a very complex and unstable one, with the same needs producing very different behaviours in different individuals.
- We all have many needs, but only a few of them are subject to conscious action at any one time.[1]

There are *intrinsic* and *extrinsic* factors at work here as well. Intrinsic factors come from within the individual, and may be positive or negative. Positive factors include wanting to succeed at something, achieving a career goal, satisfying curiosity and accepting a challenge. Such intrinsic motivational forces may be very strong.

On the other hand, extrinsic factors from outside influences include competition, respect for others, not wishing to let the side down, and admiration of one's peers. Extrinsic motivational forces may be positive or negative. Competition among students may help some but may demotivate others.

The motivational cycle

The motivational cycle is shown in Figure 8.1.

To motivate your trainees:

1   think of practical ways to motivate your learners at each session
2   make the learning interesting
3   make the learning relevant to the learners' needs
4   give regular constructive feedback on progress
5   reinforce the positive aspects and not the negative aspects of the topic and their situation
6   remember that learning feeds on success
7   give students the responsibility for learning
8   ensure that the right learning environment is provided
9   reward good performance and good discipline
10 goals should be translated into specific objectives.

Everyone likes to receive feedback and encouragement about how they are doing, so do not just leave it until the annual job appraisal, but instead give praise when and where it is due at any time.

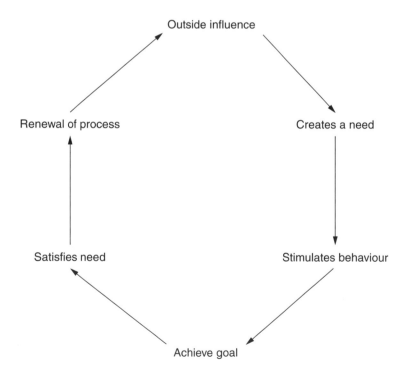

Figure 8.1:   The motivational cycle.

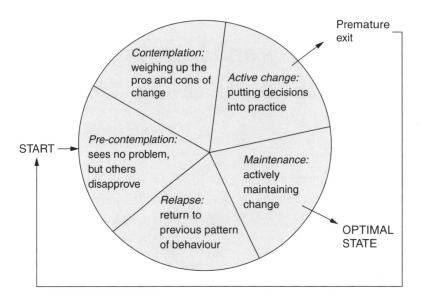

Figure 8.2:   Cycle of change.

Cycle of change[2]

The model shown in Figure 8.2 describes the stages in the cycle of change through which an individual moves, and how they must be motivated to change. It is essential to choose an appropriate time to motivate a person to change (e.g. from risky lifestyle habits to a healthy lifestyle). Individuals pass through the stage of contemplation and on to the stage of taking action for themselves. You should set realistic targets for that change which are achievable, in order to avoid demotivating the person or allowing them an escape route ('I knew I couldn't do it').

References

1   Chambers R and Wall D (2000) *Teaching Made Easy.* Radcliffe Medical Press, Oxford.

2   Prochaska J, DiClemente C and Norcross J (1992) In search of how people change. *Am Psychol.* **47**: 1102–14.

Games, activities and learning techniques

Exercise 8.1 Make up a business card to promote a new business

Why you should do this

To explore what it is that motivates those taking part in this exercise at work and in career progression or development. To realise hidden talents or interests that might remotivate the participants if they were brought to their everyday work.

When to use this

At the beginning of a day session on personal or professional development. It could be included as part of a workshop or plenary lecture format.

What to do

The participants should work in twos, threes or fours. Their task is to discuss their personal strengths and interests both in work and outside work, and then to agree what new business they could set up together if they were all to leave the health service. The new business should utilise all of their personal and professional strengths and interests. They must then design the business card using paper and coloured pens and scissors, to portray the new business and promote it to prospective clients.

The groups take turns to show each other their 'business-card' design and to explain the components and overall purpose of the business.

The groups then debrief, and each individual compares the personal and professional strengths and interests that they have just described to the others with what they currently do both at work and outside work. The discussion should centre on whether the participant, upon reflection, would wish to incorporate the strengths and interests that they are not utilising at present into their current post.

How it works (insight)

In the informal and relaxed atmosphere participants can readily describe their strengths and interests, including those that they are not currently using at work. These may serve as motivating factors to improve the individual's job satisfaction if they could be harnessed appropriately.

Whom to engage

This exercise is suitable for individuals who are feeling demoralised, who are on an updating course to maintain their day-to-day skills, or who are seeking career or personal development.

How much time you should allow

Allow at least 30 minutes for the 'getting to know each other' exercise, describing strengths and interests and formulating business plans to take account of these. Another 15 minutes should be allocated to drawing up the 'business-card' design, and a further 15 minutes for completing the discussion and review of personal strengths and interests compared with those currently employed at work.

What the facilitator should do

Establish that 'have a go' atmosphere initially. Bring plenty of paper and coloured pens.

What to do next

Encourage individuals to look at ways to incorporate at least one unused or under-used strength or interest into the duties of their current post at work. They may need to seek career counselling or negotiate with their colleagues on how to take this forward.

What makes it work better

You could have an example of 'one I prepared earlier' to give participants an idea of what is required in the way of creative thinking in relation to new business ideas and 'business-card' design.

What can go wrong

Everyone realises that they are dissatisfied in their current posts and simply leaves, rather than identifying motivating factors and seeking to enhance them in their current work.

Exercise 8.2 Draw up a force-field analysis of positive drivers and negative influences in your professional life

Why you should use this

To help people to identify and focus on the positive and negative forces in their work and/or home lives, and to gain an overview of the weighting of these factors.

When to use this

In a session on personal and professional development – as an individual or working in a group, at a workshop or by distance learning.

What to do

Participants should draw a horizontal or vertical line in the middle of a sheet of paper. Ask them to label one side 'positive' and the other side 'negative'. They should then draw arrows to represent individual positive drivers that motivate them on the positive side of the line, and negative factors that demotivate them on the negative side of the line. The thickness and length of the arrows should represent the extent of the influence – that is, a short, narrow arrow will indicate that the positive or negative factor has a minor influence, whereas a long, wide arrow will indicate a major effect. See the example in Figure 8.3 on page 90.

Participants should then take an overview of the force-field and consider whether they are content with things as they are, or whether they can think of ways to boost the positive side and minimise the negative factors. They can do this part of the exercise on their own, with a peer or a small group, or with a mentor.

How it works (insight)

This exercise helps people to realise whether a known influence in their life is a positive or negative factor. For instance, the participants may realise upon reflection that they had assumed that money in the form of a good salary was a positive motivator. However, in fact, the wish to sustain or increase their income was a negative influence on their job satisfaction, due to their inability to spend time on meaningful non-pecuniary work-related activities.

Whom to engage

The exercise is suitable for anyone and everyone at any stage in their career.

How much time you should allow

Up to an hour with ensuing discussion, and longer for subsequent action planning.

What the facilitator should do

Urge participants to subsequent action.

What to do next

Make a personal or organisational action plan to create the situations and opportunities to boost the positive factors in the participants' lives and to minimise the arrows on the negative side.

What makes it work better

Encourage the participants to invite someone who knows them well to review the force-field analysis they have drawn and to tell them honestly about any blind spots and whether they have the positive and negative influences in proportion.

What can go wrong

People may perpetuate their own misconceptions and use the force-field analysis diagram to reinforce their self-destructive behaviour in a pseudo-scientific way.

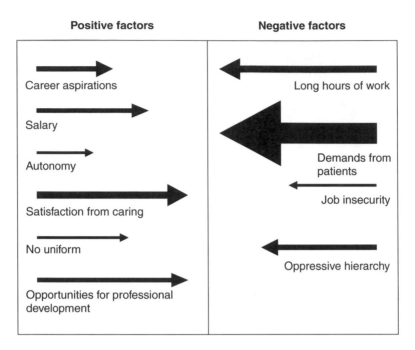

Figure 8.3:   Example of force-field analysis diagram: satisfaction with current post as a health professional.

9

Organisation of work

Increasingly people have to work in teams, and have to be managed as multidisciplinary groups at different levels. From using the skills developed in interacting in one-to-one situations we have to change to dealing with several colleagues – the people we work for and those who work for us.

Get organised as a team[1,2]

1 Review the personal development needs of the team members to fulfil their roles and responsibilities. These might relate to:
    * management skills to enable them to be effective
    * new knowledge and skills
    * their awareness of national and local policies
    * their attitudes to various subgroups of the population, or different disciplines and organisations.
2 Consider how to match the education and training resources and activities in your team with the needs of the local population.
    * Undertake a needs assessment.
    * Produce a coherent plan that embraces all of those involved.
    * Map out workforce numbers and decide whether you have the right balance.
3 Assess support needs for the individuals in your area. Plan how to allocate your resources and how to seek additional resources.
4 Encourage and enable teams to formulate and execute development plans that are centred around priority areas and include as many staff as possible.
5 Devise ways to inform and engage teams with regard to the priorities for the district and their populations. You might give practical support by supplying information or enhancing IT capability and capacity in order to make reliable and accurate data available. Summarise national documents and directives in such a way as to be useful to their everyday work.

6   Draw up a plan for the team, and allocate lines of responsibility from
     leadership to delivery. Ensure that the plan is integral to all other develop-
     mental work, such as:
     •   clinical governance
     •   monitoring performance
     •   revalidation and accreditation
     •   plans for changes to service delivery, the service and financial frame-
         work and the business and investment plan.
7   Evaluate the investment in your plan at regular intervals, and review and
     realign the priorities. Challenge historical patterns and modernise your
     approach.

Get organised as individuals

1   Staff need to be:
     •   correctly qualified to do the job when appointed *or*
     •   correctly trained to an assessed level of competence before they work
         without supervision.
2   Every staff member should have a development plan supported by the
     management.
3   Identify the education and training needs according to:
     •   the requirements of the service
     •   identified individual deficiencies in knowledge, skills or attitudes.
4   Education and training should be provided in-house or elsewhere, and
     the time to do this should be supported.

You should review your performance and that of others continuously by audit
to establish competence and identify attitude problems or gaps in knowledge
or skills.
    People carry out inappropriate tasks because:

•   they have always been done that way
•   there is no one else to do them
•   no one has thought about the best way to do them
•   they enjoy doing that job.

People who take on responsibilities outside their traditional role must ensure
that the tasks are:

•   within their personal skills and competence
•   carried out after enhancement of their knowledge or skills
•   not compromising their existing duties
•   best carried out by them and not by others with different roles or skills
•   organised so that they are able to be personally accountable for their actions.

Defining your objectives and evaluating your progress

To move forward and make improvements, you and your team need to have a clear idea of where you are heading. Establish specific objectives, agree priority topics to consider and plan your involvement or consultation exercise.[3] Set up specific targets that can be measured, so that you have some idea of how you are progressing (*see* Chapters 12, 17 and 20).

Risk management[4]

One of the most useful ways of monitoring the organisation – the process and the outcome – is by analysis of risk management. This involves:

* eliminating those risks you can get rid of
* minimising the risks you cannot eliminate
* making contingency plans for those risks that you cannot avoid.

Questions to ask before making changes:

* Is the risk large?
* Does it happen often?
* Is it a significant risk?

You do not want to spend a lot of time and effort identifying risks or making changes if they do not matter much.

Managing potential or actual risk by significant event audit

Record significant events that involved someone experiencing an adverse event or having a near miss.

1   Describe the incident.
2   Recount the effect on all of the participants.
3   Deduce the reasons for the event occurring, through discussion, review of records, procedures, etc.

4   Decide how you or others might have behaved differently, and describe your options with regard to how procedures might be changed to reduce or prevent recurrences.
5   Agree any changes that are needed, how they will be implemented, and who will be responsible for what and when.
6   Re-audit later to see whether the changes have worked. Give feedback to the team, and acknowledge good care.

Most significant incidents do not have a single cause. Usually there are faults in the system, which are compounded by one or more people being careless, tired, overworked or ill-informed. Cultivate an atmosphere of openness and discussion without blame. If people think that they will be blamed, they will hide the incident and no one will be able to prevent it from happening again. Look for *all* of the causes, and try to remedy as many as possible in order to prevent the situation from arising again. Remember that learning occurs by trying things out – fear of failure is paralysing. If we identify with an incident that happened to someone else, then we learn more as a result.

References

1   Wakley G, Chambers R and Field S (2000) *Continuing Professional Development in Primary Care: making it happen.* Radcliffe Medical Press, Oxford.
2   Chambers R and Wakley G (2000) *Making Clinical Governance Work for You.* Radcliffe Medical Press, Oxford.
3   Chambers R (2000) *Involving Patients and the Public: how to do it better.* Radcliffe Medical Press, Oxford.
4   Mohanna K and Chambers R (2001) *Risk Matters in Healthcare.* Radcliffe Medical Press, Oxford.

Games, activities and learning techniques

Exercise 9.1 Aims and contributions

Why you should do this

This activity focuses not just on what the participants hope to achieve, but also on what part they need to play in the process.

When to use this

This exercise is useful at the beginning of a session to introduce the work of the session.

What to do

Give each participant a sheet of flip-chart paper and a flip-chart pen. Ask them to draw a line across the middle about halfway down. They should head the top section 'Aims' and the bottom section 'Contributions', and put their own name at the bottom of the sheet. Ask them to write (so that others can read it) a list of their own aims for the session and what they are able and willing to contribute to the session in order to achieve them. When the time is up, give each participant a small amount of Blu-Tack and ask them to fix their sheet to the wall. Encourage everyone to walk round and read other people's sheets.

A variation of this exercise is to post each person a sheet of A4 paper similarly divided, together with brief instructions as they book on the course. The paper should be returned before the start of the course.

How it works (insight)

By writing their name on the sheet the participant 'owns' what is written, and they will think more carefully about the content. They become clearer about why they are attending the group, and they also define their role at the workshop and can see that they need to be actively involved and not just a passive observer. The lessons learned can be used in other situations.

Whom to engage

This is a useful starting point for any group, but particularly for those who need to define their aims and objectives.

How much time you should allow

Allow about five minutes for distribution of paper and pens, explaining the task and allowing each person to find enough room to write. Assign 10 minutes for the task, and another 10 to 15 minutes to fix up the sheets and read each other's responses.

What the facilitator should do

Keep time, and walk round encouraging anyone who is not getting started.

What to do next

Exercises 9.2 and 9.3 continue and refine this activity.

What makes it work better

- Participants with a clear idea of what they want from attending, and what they can do to achieve their aims.
- The aims of the participants match what is going to be provided.
- Participants write clearly so that others can read what they have written.

What can go wrong

- Participants who have been sent to the session rather than wanting to attend for themselves.
- Participants who have no clear idea what they want or what they can contribute.
- Participants who would rather remain passive.
- Participants whose writing cannot be read.
- If the information is gathered in advance, substitutes arrive for those who originally filled in the forms.
- Many of the forms may not be returned.

Exercise 9.2   Refining the aims into objectives, using the contributions

Why you should do this

It shows that you are responding to the stated aims and examining how (and if) they could be met by using the contributions of the group members and the facilitators.

When to use this

After completing Exercise 9.1, or if you have asked participants to do this in advance.

What to do

Review the sheets yourself and identify some general categories. Write these as headings on a flip chart or blank acetate sheet.

Ask each person to stand beside their sheet and in turn to read out one aim. Ask the group to provide an objective that would meet the aim, into which category it would fit, and then ask what contributions from the group members or from the facilitator would help it to be realised. Write the object-ives in one colour and the contributions in another. Add in any activities that have already been planned which meet the objectives. You will need a 'miscellaneous' category for those that do not fit neatly into any one category.

Leave the aims and objectives displayed so that you and the participants can check whether they are being met. (Be prepared to modify what you do accordingly!)

How it works (insight)

Participants can judge whether their aims are reasonable or over-ambitious and unlikely to be met by the scale of activities planned. They can recognise where their own contributions can assist with setting and meeting objectives, and where they fit in with the planned activities. They become more active participants who are less reliant on the facilitators to provide everything for them.

Whom to engage

Participants in a group or workshop who have defined their aims for a project or work programme.

How much time you should allow

This depends on the number of group members and the number of aims. Discussion usually takes about 40 to 60 minutes.

What the facilitator should do

Encourage discussion of the aims and contributions. Allow new contributions to be offered, and modification of the aims if participants realise that they are unrealistic. Try to categorise the aims and objectives as clearly as possible.

What to do next

You might use Exercise 9.3 or start on a new task.

What makes it work better

* Participants who are prepared to be flexible about what they have written down and responsible for their own learning.
* Participants who have similar aims.

What can go wrong

* Participants who cannot (or will not) recognise that their aims are unrealistic, or who cannot see that they could make any contribution towards meeting them.

- Participants with widely different aims. Also those who are unable to see how aims can be translated into objectives for learning.

Exercise 9.3   Setting priorities

Why you should do this

This exercise helps people to recognise that not everything can be covered in a learning session, and to set priorities.

When to use this

You might use this exercise after Exercise 9.2, or for any activity where there are a large number of objectives, not all of which can be met within the time or with the resources available.

What to do

List on an acetate sheet or flip chart and give a letter of the alphabet (A, B, C, etc.) to the objectives obtained either from the previous exercise or from some other activity. Ask each participant to rate each objective from 1 to 20 and to write the rating by the letter without conferring with anyone else. Explain that it is acceptable to allocate an objective '20' marks, and to rate another as 'zero', or to divide the marks more equally. Ask each group member to give you the ratings and write them alongside the objectives. Add the total rating for each objective (you may want a calculator if you get flustered when adding up quickly in public).

If there is an objective with widely different ratings, ask the participant who gave it a high rating to explain why and the person who gave it a low rating to respond to this. Allow a general discussion for each objective with different ratings.

How it works (insight)

It can be surprising for some participants to discover that items which they rated as important were not so to others. It emphasises the need to explore other people's views of what is important and to take their views into account when setting out a programme of work.

Whom to engage

Any groups that are using objectives.

How much time you should allow

This depends on the level of disagreement. If the ratings are similar, it will take about half an hour, but allow twice that time if items are hotly debated.

What the facilitator should do

Keep the peace – do not allow feelings to become too heated in defence of someone's pet idea. Move the discussion on fairly briskly to avoid spending all the time available discussing just a few of the points.

What to do next

You can use the priority ratings to give objectives to small syndicate groups. Allocate the items that they rated highly to those who are most interested in them. You might modify the content of the activities to make them more relevant to the highly rated objectives, and you could offer to set up further groups to meet the objectives that cannot be covered in the time available.

What makes it work better

Differences in the participants' views – this situation is more likely if they come from different disciplines or backgrounds.

What can go wrong

- Everyone agrees on the priorities and there is little or no discussion.
- A few participants become upset that their objectives are not rated highly by others and take it personally as a criticism of their self-worth.

Exercise 9.4 The risk rollercoaster

Why you should do this

It makes analysis of significant events more interesting and encourages lateral thinking about problem solving.

When to use this

When people are inexperienced in significant event auditing or sceptical about its value (the 'nothing ever gets done, so why bother?' attitude).

What to do

Prepare several sets of cards. Write on them situations that occur in management decisions and shuffle them well. For example, you could include the following.

1   No more money in the budget.
2   New money identified in the budget.
3   A new amount of money allocated for you to do what you want with it.
4   Your premises are a listed building.
5   Your premises are going to be upgraded.
6   Several staff members involved are moving to other posts.
7   Staff members have security of tenure because of old contracts.
8   There is resistance to change.
9   Everyone has their own different ideas about what should be done.
10   Changes have to be approved by a committee that meets quarterly.
11   The significant people are not at this meeting.
12   The records of the event have been lost.
13   The records of this event are inadequate.
14   A management directive has informed you that an example must be made of the person responsible.
15   The person involved has gone off sick with a stress-related illness.
16   The press want some information about the incident.
17   The manager has received a formal complaint.
18   A solicitor has sent a letter requesting a copy of the records for an unrelated episode.
19   The person involved has died from an unrelated event.
20   The person involved is obtaining services from another source.

Ask group members to bring their own recent significant events, and/or to provide enough examples of significant events that are relevant to the participants. You may need to make these quite general if participants come from diverse backgrounds. Health and safety items are useful in this context. For example:

- fire doors are persistently propped open
- computer wiring is dangerously situated where people can catch their clothing on it or it can be accessed by small children
- someone with a disability could not access services provided up some stairs in the building
- people living rough are rifling through the waste containers at night.

Divide into small groups, allocating participants as far as possible so that they are grouped with people with whom they do not usually work. Each group takes a significant event and a timer. One member of the group has a set of cards and the timer. Ask them to set the timer to go off after 10 minutes and then every 5 minutes. The group starts to discuss the event and the possible reasons for it. After 10 minutes they must move on to remedies for the problem. At each subsequent timer interval, the participant with the cards turns over a card and reads it out. The group then modifies what they were going to do accordingly.

Advise the group that they can leave out a card if it is repetitious and take another instead. Meet back in the plenary group to exchange experiences and have a general discussion.

How it works (insight)

This exercise helps people to treat the event as a failure of the whole system rather than of individuals. They can treat it as an exercise to be solved, and the cards encourage lateral thinking.

Whom to engage

Groups who are uncertain about the usefulness of significant event auditing, or who have rigid ways of approaching the subject.

How much time you should allow

Allow about 5 minutes for the explanation and dividing into groups, about 60 minutes for the small group work, and about 25 minutes for the exchange of views in the plenary group.

What the facilitator should do

Prepare thoroughly – you need to know in advance who is attending and their work settings so that you can provide suitable examples. Be available for disputes and encourage the group members to respond to the timer. Supply cards with typed instructions and timers that are easy to operate.

What to do next

Have a break – this is an exhausting exercise if done enthusiastically!

What makes it work better

- Amusing timers (try ones from a kitchenware or joke shop).
- Groups who can think on their feet and respond quickly to new challenges, and who are prepared to think laterally.

What can go wrong

- A group of people who think that the exercise is a waste of time, cannot see the point of trying to sort out fictional problems, and are frustrated and inhibited by their work situation.
- Rigid thinkers who find it difficult to change tack and therefore try to continue with previous solutions.

10

Leadership

The clinical leader of today works in a turmoil of change, in a resource-limited environment, helping to plot and direct the future of the workplace team or healthcare organisation. He or she has to cope with the pressures on the service from advancing technology and capability, increasing public expectations and tensions between the corporate view of the organisation and the professions' perspectives.

The range of competencies expected of clinical leaders may include the following:

- financial competency – being able to understand financial issues and ensure that business planning reflects the need to develop clinical issues; being able to manage resources
- personnel/human resources – being responsible for managing other professionals means looking after their interests and encouraging their development
- operational management – being able to co-ordinate a number of disciplines and ensure that teams work efficiently; good project management skills and the ability to use information are part of operational management
- development of strategy – being aware of the external environment, participating in the development of a vision for the organisation and contributing to the delivery of key objectives
- personal attributes – such as good time management, good communication skills, being seen as trustworthy by staff, able to negotiate, a team builder
- problem-solving and decision-making skills
- caring for the patient – having a 'customer focus' and patient-centred approach to the vision of management.

Adapted from NHS Executive (2000).[1]

Leaders in health settings[2-4]

These individuals need to have the following characteristics.

- *They develop and articulate a vision.* They understand the rationale and show how the vision can be realised. They engage people in developing the vision and reflect the vision in strategies and action.

- *They motivate others.* They design jobs so that people perform well. They invest time and energy in supporting and listening to people. They know how to motivate people and encourage high standards.
- *They make decisions.* They recognise that uncertainty and risk are part of decision making, and they seek the views and opinions of key individuals and engage others in taking decisions. They are prepared to take difficult and unpopular decisions, and they learn from and monitor the effects of previous decisions.
- *They release others' talents.* They identify and overcome barriers to individuals, teams and organisations achieving their potential. They ensure that individuals' learning and development needs are identified and met.
- *They demonstrate responsiveness and flexibility.* They are able to respond positively and competently to an unexpected event themselves, and to develop a culture of flexibility and responsiveness in the organisation as priorities change. They recognise the pressures that people are under when there is uncertainty and change.
- *They embody a set of values.* They make the values of the organisation clear to others both internally and externally, and they create respect for the people with whom they work, service users and members of the public. They work towards equity and access to services, and are good role models themselves with regard to their conduct and personal behaviour.
- *They innovate.* They encourage a culture in which creativity and innovation are welcomed and people learn from past successes or failures. They try out new ideas from both within and outside the organisation.
- *They work across boundaries.* They are committed to working in partnership and overcoming barriers to joint working (e.g. tackling professional tribalism, different structures and cultures). They create opportunities for joint working, and can negotiate with partner organisations to minimise conflicting priorities.
- *They demonstrate resilience and assistance.* They not only demonstrate self-confidence themselves, but also build confidence in individuals and teams. They develop strategies to avoid burnout in the workforce, and have insight into their own and others' strengths and weaknesses.

References

1   NHS Executive (2000) *Workforce Development and Building Leadership in the NHS.* NHS Executive, London.

2   Frances D and Woodcock M (1996) *The Unblocked Manager.* Gower, Aldershot.

3   Scott T (2000) Clinicians in management. In: *Leadership in Health: a UK perspective on clinical leadership. Part 2. Healthcare Review Online*™. **4**: February.

4   Simpson J (2000) Clinical leadership in the UK. In: *Leadership in Health: a UK perspective on clinical leadership. Part 2. Healthcare Review Online*™. **4**: February.

Games, activities and learning techniques

Exercise 10.1 An opportunity in the car park: making an impact

Why you should use this

To encourage participants to think creatively in a pressured situation.

When to use this

In a workshop to encourage leadership in teams, and to improve communication skills.

What to do

People work in pairs and perform this role-play exercise in front of the other participants. One member of the pair plays the role of a senior member of an organisation (e.g. the chief executive), and the other member plays a junior manager. The remit of the junior manager is to engage the senior manager in a conversation and generate interest in a particular project. The junior manager has up to two minutes to interest his or her senior before they head off for an important meeting – to the extent that the senior person will want to meet again and discuss the idea further. Each participant should then give feedback to the other to say how the scene felt, whether they thought that their interest had been sufficiently stirred to agree to meet at a later date, etc.

The subsequent discussion should cover the feelings of both participants as a pair. The plenary group can then share their experiences and swap techniques that can be used to make an appropriate impact.

The types of topics that might be of interest could include buying new equipment, a lack of facilities or administrative support in the department, developing a partnership with another organisation, or producing a poster or a newsletter.

How it works (insight)

This exercise mimics real life. It allows individual participants to think creatively and consider their issue from the senior person's perspective. The role play also allows participants to explore what pressured situations feel like, and to develop techniques for dealing with such stress.

Whom to engage

Any participants with an interest in leadership, management, communication techniques and/or creative thinking.

How much time you should allow

Up to 30 minutes for four or five role-play exercises, and a further 20 to 40 minutes for discussion, depending on the size of the group.

What the facilitator should do

Set the scene and explain the aims of the junior manager. The facilitator must also ensure that the senior person breaks off conversation after two minutes.

What to do next

Encourage individuals to make personal action plans that build on the role-play experience to address any weaknesses or acquire further skills. Run follow-up sessions on communication techniques, assertiveness skills, etc.

What makes it work better

Creating as realistic an atmosphere as possible – for example, by encouraging participants who are playing the junior manager's role to use real-life pet topics that they would like to promote.

What can go wrong

- The role play might be taken too seriously, or the participants playing the junior manager might end up in conflict with the senior role player.
- Some participants might be reluctant to 'perform' in front of the plenary group.
- Some of the less creative participants or those who are hostile to role play may find it difficult to think of a topic that is potentially interesting enough, or may refuse to join in the exercise.

Exercise 10.2 Heroes and heroines

Why you should do this

To identify important skills and characteristics required in leadership roles that are relevant to the participants. To magnify the importance of these skills and characteristics by identifying with heroes or heroines.

When to use this

In a group session covering leadership roles, or on a leadership programme.

What to do

1 Split the large group into smaller teams of about five or six people.
2 Ask the teams to identify one leadership role which is relevant to at least some of the participants (e.g. clinical team leader, primary care team leader, departmental head, director, etc.).
3 Ask the teams to identify key attributes, skills and characteristics required of such a role, and to list these (e.g. introducing change, bringing out the best in people, creating a vision, etc.).
4 Taking each skill or attribute in turn, ask the team members to identify well-known characters (these could be living, or historical, fictional or non-fictional) who could illustrate each of the skills or attributes on the list.
5 Feed back to the plenary group with a list of skills and characters.

How it works (insight)

It allows people to reflect on what is required in leadership roles, and then to illustrate these requirements in a visual way.

Whom to engage

Those engaged or aspiring to engage in leadership roles.

How much time you should allow

Allow 10 minutes for identifying the list of key skills or attributes, 30 minutes for identifying characters, and a further 20 to 40 minutes to feed back and develop a composite list of attributes and heroes or heroines in the plenary group.

What the facilitator should do

Explain the purpose of the exercise and ensure that all members of the team can contribute towards developing a list of attributes and associated characters, and explain why these have been selected.

What to do next

Ask individuals to identify which of the attributes and skills they wish to develop further, and make plans with regard to how this can be achieved.

What makes it work better

The facilitator should be able to cite examples of instantly recognisable role models when explaining the 'rules' of the exercise.

What can go wrong

- Participants may lack creative skills and find it difficult to think of heroes or heroines.
- Participants may be overawed at the conclusion by the qualities required for the particular role in question. Emphasise that in real life all of the skills and attributes would not be present in any one person. They are merely personal qualities to which to aspire.

Exercise 10.3 Appointment with the boss

Why you should do this

This exercise can be used to promote listening and analytical feedback, as well as for developing creative solutions.

When to use this

This should ideally be used well into a workshop (e.g. on the second day). If it is used very early on, ask the participants to identify suitable problems before they come to the workshop.

What to do

1 Participants should define a particular work problem which is easy to describe and understand in one or two minutes.

2   Divide the participants into equal numbers of 'leaders' and 'workers', and try to ensure a good mixing of participants. If there are enough people, divide leaders and workers into A and B teams. Workers and leaders work together in the first round.

3   The leaders are sited in an 'office' which consists of two chairs at a reasonable distance from the next office.

4   Each 'A' worker spends 10 minutes with each 'B' leader in his or her 'office' describing their particular problem and discussing possible solutions. Both leaders and workers make notes on the problem and on the solutions that emerge.

5   Workers then rotate to the next 'office' and describe the same problem with a different leader.

6   Once the 'A' workers have consulted three 'B' leaders, the roles are reversed. 'A' workers become leaders and work with 'B' leaders (who become workers), and vice versa. The exercise is repeated with the new roles.

7   Following this, there is a discussion of the different consulting styles, approaches and solutions that emerged from the consultations.

How it works (insight)

This exercise allows participants to act as leaders and use their skills to help workers to develop solutions. The workers gain insight into the various approaches that may be applied to the same problem, and the variety of solutions that emerge.

Whom to engage

This exercise works best with no more than 10 to 12 people who would like to develop leadership, listening and analytical skills.

How much time you should allow

Allow 60 minutes for the consultations and 30 to 60 minutes for the subsequent discussions.

What the facilitator should do

Give the participants adequate warning to enable them to prepare suitable problems. Strict timekeeping is important. When the roles are reversed, if possible the new workers should consult different leaders to those whom they met previously when they were role-playing leaders. The facilitator should describe best practice in listening, consulting skills and feedback before the exercise begins, and this should be reinforced during the discussion.

What to do next

This exercise could serve as a platform for more group-based problem solving and decision making.

What makes it work better

Instead of working as pairs, an observer might be one of a trio, sitting in and making notes and giving independent feedback.

What can go wrong

- There may be insufficient time for sensible solutions to emerge.
- Some of the problems that are presented may be inappropriate for this type of session (e.g. a complex clinical problem or a highly technical problem relating to information technology).

11

Strategy

In simple terms, a strategy involves defining an overall goal and developing a plan to achieve that goal.

The key components of development of a strategy include the following:

- developing a vision or goal(s)
- understanding the current environment
- planning
- managing change
- leadership.

Developing a vision

A vision needs to be embedded in reality – otherwise there is a danger of it becoming more of a hallucination! A clear, shared vision of the future can be useful for shaping change. Questions that can help to develop a vision of the future may include the following.

- What are the major trends in society and how will these affect our organisation?
- What will our customers/stakeholders require of us in five years' time?
- What will happen if we stay as we are?
- What critical events that are likely to occur in the future will affect us?

This vision outlines the core purpose of the organisation and its reason for existence.

Understanding the environment

A key element of developing a strategy is mapping out the current environment. All of the influences on the organisation and the individuals within it need to be considered, including the following:

- government bodies
- pressure groups

- media
- consumers
- suppliers
- research
- laws
- policies
- information, etc.

It is important to understand the key influences and how they affect the behaviour of the organisation both now and in the future.

Management of the strategy

The logical approach to managing the strategy and creating change is as follows.

1 Develop a strategy.
2 Produce a plan.
3 Seek approval.
4 Implement the strategy.

However, experience shows that this process rarely works. In reality, programmes of change are more complex and occur through different sequences of the above steps.

When a strategy goes wrong ...

Many a health service strategy gathers dust on a bookshelf for one or more of the following reasons.

It is not read or understood

Once a strategy has been produced, it needs to be seen, read and understood by the target audience. Careful thought needs to be given to how the message should be communicated to key movers and shakers.

It is too vague and woolly

An implementation plan with targets and milestones is essential.

It is too prescriptive

A strategy which is too detailed and lacks flexibility may not meet local needs, and may therefore fail.

It lacks ownership

An essential element of strategy development should be to engage key players, including consumers/patients.

Unexpected events occur

Unexpected events (e.g. a new government initiative) can blow a strategy off course. The strategy should be flexible to enable it to adapt to new circumstances.

It is launched at the wrong time

The timing can be wrong for an otherwise perfect strategy – it may be ahead of its time or too late. It is perfectly reasonable to develop a strategy and wait for the right time for its implementation.

The financial implications

With many competing priorities for scarce health service resources, a strategy should assess the financial implications and ensure that appropriate resources are secured.

Has it worked?

It may not be possible to answer this question unless mechanisms for evaluating progress are established at an early stage.

Games, activities and learning techniques

Exercise 11.1 Lightning strikes three times

Why you should do this exercise

For participants to learn to devise a strategy to tackle a relevant problem.

When to use this

Once participants are familiar with some of the theory of developing strategy.

What to do

1   The facilitator divides the participants into groups of seven or eight people and asks them to select (or allocates) one of the problem options.
2   Each small group is given a different problem.
3   The following roles are allocated within each group by giving each person a written description of their role:
    *   a *leader* whose job is to set goals and ensure that decisions are made
    *   an *expert* who has technical skills relevant to the problem
    *   a *challenger* who can challenge ideas and current presumptions
    *   a *finance manager* who is in charge of financial matters for the organisation
    *   a *visionary* who can focus on the organisation ahead and form beliefs of what it is capable of and what it should be achieving in the future
    *   an *operational manager* whose job is to get things done and develop ways of making sure that they happen
    *   a *teambuilder* who binds the various strengths and weaknesses of group members and helps them to work towards common objectives
    *   a *customer* who can give feedback to the organisation.
4   The group's task is to develop a strategy for the future to tackle current and future problems that the organisation might face. The group members should decide where they are now in their role, where they need to be in the future and how they will get there.
5   Once each group has finalised their strategy, they take turns to present their plans to the other groups for a constructive critique.

How it works (insight)

The arbitrary problem allows the group members to practise on an achievable task to master skills in developing strategy, before they are faced with more complex problems in the real world.

Whom to engage

This exercise is suitable for senior and middle managers within the health field who are involved in decision making and would like to enhance their skills for tackling problems and developing long-term solutions.

How much time you should allow

Around an hour should be allowed to develop the strategies for three groups of seven to eight people. Around 40 minutes should be allowed for 5- to 10-minute presentations with ensuing discussion and feedback.

What the facilitator should do

The facilitator should provide appropriate problem scenarios and background information with regard to the nature of the participating organisations.

Provide labels for each individual describing their role (e.g. leader, team-builder, etc.). There should be adequate materials (e.g. flip charts, overhead projector sheets, pens, papers, etc.) available.

What to do next

Future sessions could cover how the process of developing strategy went, what the most useful roles were and what they contributed, and how the approaches that were taken could be improved.

What makes it work better

Interesting roles and descriptions.

What can go wrong

- People not being willing to play the role that has been allocated to them.
- If the descriptions of the various roles are not written down, the participants may forget the details and mix components of several roles into one, causing confusion. People may drop their role and be themselves.

Some typical problems are listed below.

Problem A
A five-doctor general practice in a deprived area finds that:

- the computer system that was bought a year ago is still in storage
- there is a very rapid turnover of administrative and support staff and high rates of absenteeism. One of the GP partners is on long-term sick leave
- it has been told by the primary care trust that it is not meeting National Service Framework targets.

Problem B
A successful pharmaceutical company finds that:

- there is a serious legal challenge from patient groups. If the company loses this, it would cost it millions of pounds
- many competitors are challenging its leading drug
- share prices on the stock-market are falling drastically.

Problem C

An elderly care department in an acute hospital trust has found that:

*   there are ongoing conflicts between the consultants in the department and also between this department and the general medicine department
*   the Royal College of Physicians is threatening to withdraw accreditation because of concern about training standards for junior doctors
*   an audit has shown that the care of stroke patients is substandard because of the lack of a stroke unit.

Exercise 11.2 The 'A' team

Why you should do this

To learn more about teambuilding and strategy development.

When to use this

This is a complex exercise and individuals will need to be reasonably familiar with other members of the workshop. It is probably best undertaken in the latter half of a workshop.

What to do

Divide participants into teams of four to five people. Give the teams a series of options and ask them to choose a challenge and then produce an action plan. A series of options could include the following:

*   establishing a recruitment agency
*   developing a computer-servicing business
*   developing a new primary care team
*   developing a new clinical directorate.

The group members should identify the skills, knowledge, experience and strengths of individual members of the team and compare these with the attributes required to meet the chosen objective. Finally, they should present the action plan to the plenary group, describing how individuals will contribute.

How it works (insight)

This exercise gives participants an opportunity to practise and reflect in a fictional situation where there are no real-life consequences.

Whom to engage

People on strategy and leadership training courses or who are learning about teambuilding.

How much time you should allow

Up to 60 minutes should be allocated for the teams to produce their action plans, and then 5–10 minutes for each team to present their case. Thus for four teams you should allow 60–100 minutes in total.

What the facilitator should do

The facilitator should identify a set of objectives which are relevant to the participants. Supply appropriate materials, such as flip-chart pens, and assess the progress of the groups, checking that they select their topics promptly and get on with producing action plans.

What to do next

Debrief and plan future sessions around participants' capabilities at drawing up action plans and their development needs.

What makes it work better

The objectives need to capture the imagination of the teams.

What can go wrong

- Teams may spend too long selecting topics, so give them a 5-minute deadline for this stage.
- Teams may run out of time.
- Some teams may be totally dysfunctional and have little output. This might lead to recriminations between individual team members, especially if there are personality conflicts.

Exercise 11.3 Pennies in a box: the Delphi technique*

Why you should do this

The Delphi technique is commonly used by many organisations to obtain consensus decisions involving complex issues. The exercise also allows participants to discuss their feelings and pressures when involved in decision making.

---

* Dalkey NC (1969) *The Delphi Method: an experimental study of group opinion*. Rand Corporation, Santa Monica, CA.

When to use this

To demonstrate different approaches to decision making.

What to do

Place a tin of coins in front of all the participants, who are then free to examine the tin of coins by holding and shaking the container. Each participant should write down the number of coins that they think are present. The facilitator then collates all of these numbers and writes them on the board. The discussion that follows considers why people suggested a particular number, and the people who guessed the fewest and the most pennies are encouraged to justify their positions. Individuals are then asked to guess again the number of coins in the tin. Discussion follows as to why participants changed their estimates (if they did so), and the process is repeated a third time. The means of each of the three sets of guesses are then compared with the actual number of coins in the tin.

How it works (insight)

With the Delphi technique a set of experts are posed a question (they do not necessarily have to be together at the same time, i.e. it could be done by telephone, post, etc.). Their responses are summarised and fed back to the individuals either anonymously or on a named basis, depending on the issue. The individual participants then have an opportunity to modify their responses in the light of the answers given by other individuals and the process is repeated. There may be two, three or four rounds. Opinions tend to converge so that there is a greater degree of consensus in the final rounds.

Whom to engage

This particular technique can be used in a workshop with six or more people.

How much time you should allow

The process should be completed in about 30 minutes.

What the facilitator should do

Prepare a tin containing a large known number of coins before the meeting. Explain the process, encourage discussion, write down all of the scores on a board, and calculate the means for each round (take a calculator!).

What to do next

Participants should discuss how this method could be used in decision making within their organisation and give examples. They could debate the strengths and weaknesses of this approach.

What makes it better

A range of other alternatives could be used for the expert opinion (e.g. estimating the length of a table, height of a door, etc.).

What can go wrong

People may not change their views after the first estimate – but this rarely happens.

12

Managing change

Look at the flow chart in Figure 12.1 to see how people react to change.

We start off by being taken by surprise about a change, even if we have anticipated it. There is still a shock element when it first occurs and we are not quite sure what has happened. We move from that shock to pretending that it is not going to happen.

After the denial phase in the change process we move on to find somebody to blame for what has happened – and we tend to blame the messengers who announce the change. After the blame comes self-blame.

Part of the next stage, the bargaining, is negotiating that if we do it *this* way we are going to be able to do *that*. Eventually we arrive at the resolution phase where we have accepted the change.

We pass through these different stages of change according to how we are as people. When change is imposed on us we are very much more resistant to it, so we move more slowly. If the effect of the change is serious, our feelings about it will be stronger and we spend longer in the denial, blame and self-blame phases.[1]

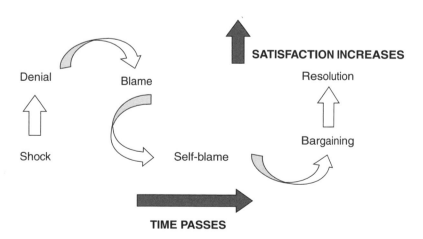

Figure 12.1: Stages of the response to change.

Planning change

We need to identify clearly the causes of dissatisfaction with the present situation, and then have a clear idea of where to head for. Map out how to reach that target, and find the way in staged steps to measure progress towards the target.

Identifying the barriers and problems[2]

People play roles in response to change. For example:

- the rebel – 'I don't see why I should'
- the victim – 'I suppose you will make me, but I will drag my feet'
- the oppressor – 'You all have to do it'
- the rescuer – 'I will save you all from this terrible change'.

Therefore the following points are important.

- Have realistic time-scales and be flexible.
- Provide clear communication about what is happening.
- Consult with all of the staff, identifying all of the problems as they occur.
- Plan for more resources and time than you expect to use.
- Fix interval markers of progress.
- Feed the information about what is happening back to people.
- Identify the anxieties and try to resolve them.
- Consider the effects of this change on other services and people.
- Beware of too many changes taking place at once.
- Recognise that change can be hijacked by vested interests and its direction altered.
- Be prepared to change direction if necessary.
- Beware of a lack of commitment from others.

Managing change within organisations

The process of managing transition differs in many ways from managing current and routine business. The change process itself requires different styles of management, different organisational structures (in particular, a lot of project-based work) and different skills.

Organisations that are undergoing change often appoint project managers, and project teams are formed which include representatives from the groups that are most involved in change to gain ownership of the change process. A common mistake that organisations make is to give existing managers the responsibility for managing change. These managers do not necessarily have the time or the right skills, and are often operating systems which are suited to the present state rather than the desired one.

Management of change invariably requires investment of resources in the short term.

References

1   Upton T and Brooks B (1995) *Managing Change*. Open University Press, Buckingham.

2   Riley J (1998) *Helping Doctors Who Manage*. King's Fund Publishing, London.

Games, activities and learning techniques

Exercise 12.1 Writing the play

Why you should do this

To identify more clearly the roles and strategies that people adopt when faced with change, and to look at ways of managing people so that necessary change is not thwarted.

When to use this

In a workshop after a talk or large-group interactive session on managing change, so that the participants come to understand the principles for themselves. You might use it with a group that is just starting to look at ways of managing change, or with a group that has already run into difficulties with a project.

What to do

Divide into small groups of four to six participants. Ask them to write a short play incorporating the roles of victim, oppressor, rescuer and rebel, as well as any other hidden agendas that they think appropriate. A recorder and an analyst should be nominated in each group and supplied with a pad of paper or a flip chart and pens. The flip chart should be divided into two unequal columns, with the wider one on the left. Ask the recorder to write the play in the left-hand column. When hidden agendas or role playing are identified in the behaviour of the actors by any member of the group, the analyst should record this in the right-hand column.

There are two options. First, a ready-made scenario such as the following can be provided.

1   The committee of a voluntary group is discussing whether to become involved in a protest about changes proposed to close several elderly care homes and increase the funding for keeping people in their own homes. One of them is a relative of an elderly person who will have to move when her elderly care home is closed. Another works for social services and is aware of the under-occupancy and high running costs of the home. A third committee member is a vehement supporter of care at home, while a fourth wants to use the protest to gain publicity for the voluntary society.

2   An extended family with parents, teenage and young single adult offspring, grandparents and aunts is discussing what to do if the mushroom factory in the community closes, as is rumoured will happen. Most people in the community work at the factory or in supporting activities. The parents and two of the young adults in the family work at the factory, one young adult works in the office, one aunt at the school and one grandparent at the local shop and café next to the factory.

Alternatively, ask each group to choose a scenario from their own experience or current knowledge. You might use Exercise 12.2 ('Having a moan') in a prior session in order to identify changes that they feel need to be made.

How it works (insight)

The process of writing the dialogue (to illustrate the roles and hidden agendas that people have when faced with a change) crystallises the identification of those hidden or open agendas. It makes it easier to be aware of the difficulties that people may be experiencing in accepting or making changes. Using the interchange of dialogue between fictitious characters allows experimentation with strategies to manage change better.

The use of art, such as writing a play in this instance, acts as a stimulus which takes participants out of their work contexts, and can seem less threatening than traditional learning approaches.

Whom to engage

A group of staff members of varying seniority working together on a project that is experiencing difficulties.

People attending a course on managing change, or individuals who have identified that they will have to manage change as part of an action plan that has already been drawn up.

How much time you should allow

Allow 10 minutes to give names to the actors and list their roles and allegiances, 50 minutes to write the dialogue, and 30 minutes to review and discuss what has been written, and to finish identifying and recording all of the roles and strategies in a systematic way. That is, you should allow about 90 minutes in total.

What the facilitator should do

Help the group to define or choose their scenario if they are in difficulties. Remind the groups about timekeeping. Intervene with suggestions if the group becomes stuck for ideas.

What to do next

Reconvene in the plenary group. Ask the members for feedback on drawing analogies between the roles and strategies identified in the 'play' and examples from their work or other experience. Offer to send a typed copy of the 'play' to group members if they would like one. If they want copies, ask them to record their names on the 'play' script.

What makes it work better

- Using a fictional or non-personal example often liberates people to be more imaginative.
- Using a scenario with relevance to the group's working experience makes it more realistic.
- Using this exercise in a group where people feel able to be creative and uninhibited.

What can go wrong

- A newly formed group that is not at ease finds it difficult to be creative – members are afraid of 'making a fool of themselves'.
- Using this exercise in a staff group that is very hierarchical – junior staff may fear disapproval if they put their ideas forward.
- A group of participants that is mainly composed of very practical, active or pragmatic learners will find it difficult to identify behaviours that are hidden.
- The group may be taken over by one person who fancies him- or herself as a playwright and extinguishes other people's suggestions with scorn.

Exercise 12.2 Having a moan

Why you should do this

It enables the participants to identify areas of dissatisfaction and to see them as issues that require solutions. It makes clear the necessity to know what needs changing before proposing change. It helps to start the process of setting a goal and knowing how to get there.

When to use this

If there is an undercurrent of complaint and dissatisfaction, either with the workshop, or with the work situation from which the participants have come.

What to do

This exercise can be organised in several ways:

- in pairs – exchanging moans and discussing them, trying to come up with solutions. Each pair then presents the moans and solutions to the whole group
- the whole group brainstorms all of the moans without discussion, and then ranks them into priorities. The group then proposes solutions to some of the higher-priority matters
- if the group is large, divide into smaller groups (8 to 10 people) to do the above exercise
- anonymous moans are written down and put in a box. The facilitator pulls them out one by one and writes on the flip chart the solutions proposed by the group
- moans are written on 'post-it' notes. In discussion with the group, the facilitator categorises them into related themes. Group members then propose solutions for each cluster of moans.

How it works (insight)

This exercise makes the link between identifying a problem and proposing a solution. It can identify how trivial some of the moans are and how easily they can be rectified once they have been examined. The exercise can also identify some very difficult and possibly insoluble problems that have to be tolerated.

Whom to engage

Any group in which underlying dissatisfaction is recognised.

How much time you should allow

You should aim to allow only enough time for each person to state or write down the problem – perhaps 3 to 5 minutes, and then 10 to 15 minutes for the solutions and discussion. If you feed the problems and solutions back to a plenary group, allow 5 minutes for reporting and 5 minutes for further group discussion.

What the facilitator should do

Come prepared with some examples of problems in case people are reticent, especially at first.

Keep tight control of the timing, have legible writing, and ensure that everyone has an opportunity to have their say. Be prepared for criticism of the workshop, and open to discussion of how it might be run differently to meet the needs of the participants. Be prepared to act on the proposed solutions if they are possible, or to give feedback to the organisers of the workshop if not.

What to do next

You could use this session to feed into the previous exercise. You might ask the participants to make changes, or an action plan, before the next workshop to work towards the solutions proposed. If there is no follow-up session, ask the participants to write on a postcard what changes they will have made by three months from the date of the workshop. This can be posted to them when three months have elapsed, to remind them of the changes they were going to make (*see* Exercise 17.1).

What makes it work better

- A comfortable atmosphere in which group participants can reveal what they feel.
- Problems that are clearly identified.
- Enough and varied problems to make it interesting.

What can go wrong

- Fear of voicing discontent, especially in groups where managers and the staff whom they manage are present.
- Such a sense of disillusionment that there is felt to be no point in complaining, as nothing ever gets changed.

- Lack of clarity in the complaints, so that the point at issue cannot be identified.
- Too many areas of complaint, so that people feel that 'their' problem has not had an adequate hearing.
- Too many insoluble moans that make the group members feel depressed and hopeless.

13

Organisational management

The results of good organisational management will be high standards of performance from happy, well-motivated staff. The organisation should function appropriately at all levels for the quality of its outputs (care and services in the health service) to be assured.

The way to achieve continuous improvement in performance is by the organisation adopting a developmental approach that encourages staff, rather than issuing 'top-down' directives that are resented by staff and difficult to implement.

Everyone working in the practice or health service unit should be clear about the goals, individuals' roles and responsibilities, the timetabled programmes for improvements and the standards of performance required.

The three components of good organisational management are:

- people
- environment
- process.

People

Consider the number of skilled and experienced staff that you will need in order to deliver your vision of care and services. Concentrate on building up cohesive teams that function effectively under good leadership. Create the environment and processes within the organisation that breed well-motivated staff with high levels of job satisfaction.

Environment

The environment includes the physical structure of the premises and contents, and the technical capacity, such as medical equipment and IT hardware and software. Regular and thorough risk assessment, followed by risk reduction and monitoring, are essential aspects of good organisational management of the workplace environment.

Process

The process includes policies, procedures and systems. Good organisational management of the process of planning and delivering care and services will reduce the likelihood of mistakes occurring. Errors will be picked up by failsafe systems before there is any opportunity for harm. Good process will ensure that staff only undertake activities in which they are competent. Well-disseminated policies enable everyone in the workplace to know how systems and procedures work, and give consistent messages to patients.

The results

An essential feature of good organisational management will be measuring the performance of the organisation and feeding this back to plan for continuous improvement. Measures might focus on the effectiveness and efficiency of the delivery of care, and access to health services by various subgroups of the patient population. Both patients' and staff's reports of their experiences should be used to readjust systems and procedures to improve the quality of care and services provided. This might be qualitative (e.g. from individual complaints or focus group discussions) or quantitative (e.g. from a sampled population survey).

A positive culture will include regular feedback to staff about performance, clear leadership, good communication, well-organised services, and encouragement for each individual member of staff.

Understanding the formal and informal features of an organisation may help staff to adapt and fit into the way in which their employing organisation operates. Formal and informal features have an equally important influence on the nature of an organisation and on the happiness and productivity of staff.

The formal features of an organisation are as follows:

- organisation of hierarchies and accountability arrangements
- committee structures
- meetings
- information systems
- arrangements for financial controls
- pay and reward
- monitoring systems, etc.

The informal features of an organisation are as follows:

- culture of the organisation
- relationships

- honesty
- extent of game playing
- teamwork
- how people work
- effectiveness of communication
- real distribution of power
- conflicts and how these are handled
- informal rewards.

Equity

Equity is an important end-point that can be used as a measure of how well the organisation is managed.

For staff, equity might concern the following:

- equal access to opportunities for staff development
- equal treatment with regard to least favourite duties (e.g. covering public holidays)
- allowances for those with disabilities (e.g. special chairs)
- staff who work in branch surgeries or peripheral clinics not being dis-advantaged.

For patients, equity at practice level might concern the following:

- a range of appropriate services available in the practice for all age groups
- facilities for disabled people
- opening hours that are convenient for all
- special arrangements for access for homeless people.

For doctors, equity with medical colleagues might concern the following:

- distribution of workload between doctors and other health professionals in the workplace
- financial shares of doctors
- proportional share of responsibilities
- democratic decision making.

Source of information

Much of the material in this chapter was derived from the presentation by Mr P Griffiths, Chief Executive of Health Quality Service, at the conference on 'Involving patients and the public in primary care' in Birmingham in May 2001.

Games, activities and learning techniques
Exercise 13.1 Talking walls

Why you should use this

To help members of mixed teams to understand others' perspectives or responsibilities, and to brainstorm about the scope of topic areas (problems, solutions, etc.).

When to use this

This technique has been used successfully in undergraduate education of medical, dental, nursing and therapy students, and in the continuing professional development of primary care teams.

What to do

Individuals list their perceptions about a variety of topics on flip-chart sheets (one per topic) displayed on the walls of the workshop room. The types of topics you might use for this include the following:

- about people: teambuilding
- about the working environment: perceived risks and assumptions
- about process: patients' experiences.

Learners contribute to each sheet, describing their views about all of the topics except any topic(s) that relate to them or on which they are experts. Once the lists are complete, the learners examine the topic(s) in which they have expertise and indicate with a different coloured pen any misconceptions, inaccuracies and omissions.

The ensuing discussion enables each group member to clarify confusion and misunderstanding about the contents of the lists (in the example situation given above, individuals' roles or experiences or the constraints of their jobs).

How it works (insight)

Everyone is engaged in contributing their ideas in a non-threatening way – input is not attributed to individuals. This exercise utilises the expertise of particular members of the team which might not normally be acknowledged in everyday life.

Whom to engage

Use this exercise for small mixed groups of participants. For example, an inter-professional group might consider the roles, responsibilities or experiences of the different professions involved in the exercise, and a practice team might explore their perceptions of stressors and stress management.

How much time you should allow

This will depend on the number of topics you are working on and how complex they are. Allow 15 minutes for the initial brainstorming, and up to 15 minutes for the various experts to make their corrections. Then take each topic page by page to discuss the reasons for the variation in views between the participants and the 'expert'. This last section may take over an hour if there are three or four topics and the group debates the ways forward and the barriers to progress, so allow two hours in total.

What the facilitator should do

Make the exercise come alive for the participants – it is not simply another activity with headings and lists. Identify the relevant topics and the topic 'experts' among the participants. Remind the experts not to contribute to those topics at the initial brainstorming stage. Encourage an informal atmosphere in which the expert input is given in an informative and non-judgemental way.

Draw the exercise to a positive conclusion with a useful ending that paves the way for subsequent action planning and application of change.

What to do next

Agree a consensus outlook on each topic area where there was previous disagreement or disparity. This could be formally ratified as a workplace policy or protocol, or by the introduction of new systems and procedures.

What makes it work better

- Topics that are relevant to as many participants as possible.
- An alternative version is for the participants or the facilitator to write on separate pieces of paper nouns or short phrases that are connected with the theme of the learning event to develop a conceptual model. These are

attached to the wall with Blu-Tack. The participants then move the nouns or short phrases around the wall and connect them to each other with lines. After discussion, the learners suggest and agree on verbs that link the nouns or short phrases to make a flow path. For instance, if the topic was diabetes, and nouns such as 'blood sugar', 'hypertension', 'complications' and 'well-being' were displayed, all of these words could be linked to each other, and verbs such as 'reduce', 'minimise' or 'increase' could be considered.*

What can go wrong

The mixed group of participants should hold diverse views, as the whole exercise will be pointless if everyone is in agreement from the start.

Exercise 13.2 Timetable tasks with a Gantt chart

Why you should use this

To help participants to understand how to make a timetabled plan for improving the management of a service that they currently provide, or to set up a new service.

When to use this

This exercise is suitable for an interactive workshop or small group work with individuals from different organisations or the same organisation (e.g. a practice, trust, or primary care organisation).

What to do

- *Stage 1*: The facilitator asks the participants to shout out all the aspects of the organisational management that they would have to think of in order to set up a new (clinical) service. These are noted down on a flip chart as they are suggested. When the ideas have dried up, the flip chart(s) are displayed so that all of the participants can refer to them.
- *Stage 2*: The participants then work in small groups to design the pathway in the order that jobs should be tackled and sustained in order to achieve a well-organised and well-managed service, using a Gantt chart (*see* page 137 for an example).

---

* This exercise has been adapted from Pritchard P and Hughes J (1995) *Shared Care*. Nuffield Trust, London.

- *Stage 3*: Two groups meet together and compare their Gantt charts. In particular, they look at the range and type of factors that they have considered, and the timing of each aspect. At this stage the original groups are free to add new features to their Gantt charts and to change the timing.
- *Stage 4*: An expert in organisational management then visits the session. The expert gives a talk on organisational management with regard to setting up a new service.
- *Stage 5*: The groups again review their individual Gantt charts and decide whether they wish to extend their contents to add new factors or change the timing of activities.
- *Stage 6*: Finally, the expert reviews the individual Gantt charts and comments on how well thought out they are in the light of his or her own experience.

How it works (insight)

The participants should move along a spectrum of learning about organisational management from Stage 2 (as above), when they define their initial plans from their own knowledge, to Stage 3, when discussion with others may broaden their horizons, to Stage 4, when they have the opportunity to listen to the expert and consider where their plans are lacking in comparison, to Stage 5, when discussion with others confirms these gaps, and Stage 6, when there is an expert review.

The Gantt chart is a useful planning aid for a project. It can be used to calculate project activities for the total expected duration of the project. In doing this, it forces the project team to identify all of the activities that will be involved at any particular time, and to ensure that they have sufficient resources.

Whom to engage

This is an exercise for novices to organisational management (e.g. clinicians).

How much time you should allow

Allow at least an hour to give time for discussion. The total amount of time will depend on how complex the new service will be, and how long a talk the expert gives.

What the facilitator should do

Demonstrate how to make a Gantt chart. Show the participants how this can be produced on a computer or by drawing by hand.

What to do next

Encourage the participants to put their new-found knowledge into practice by making a timetabled activity plan for a new service development or an intended change to a service.

What makes it work better

- The right expert who is content to stand back and let the participants work through their planning stages.
- Ask people in the present organisation to report a few current problems with the management. Test out whether the new plan is designed to deal proactively with these particular problems.

What can go wrong

- The participants may be reluctant to explore their lack of knowledge and skills when an expert will be lecturing on the subject later, and might not co-operate with the initial part of the exercise using their current knowledge and skills in organisational management.
- Non-managers (e.g. clinicians) may not be interested in learning about organisational management because they do not consider that management is their responsibility, or they assume that they know all about it without being formally taught.

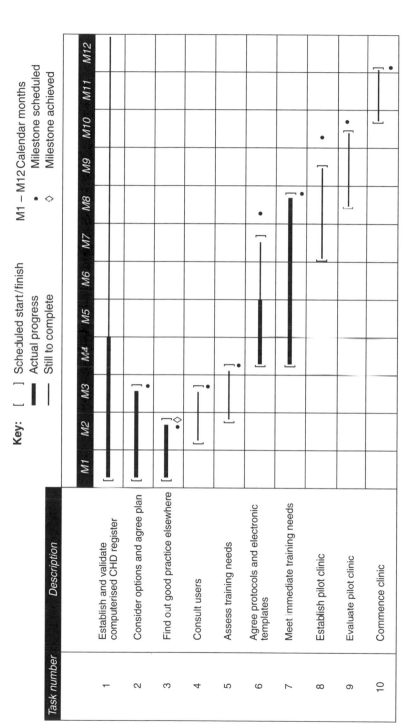

Figure 13.1:   Example of a Gantt chart: setting up a nurse-led coronary heart disease (CHD) secondary prevention clinic.

14

Time management

The many ways to manage your time better fall into three main categories:

1 *reducing the amount of work to be done* by refusing it in the first place, delegating it, or doing less of it
2 *doing the work more quickly* by doing it less thoroughly or processing it more efficiently
3 *allowing more time for the particular piece of work* so that there is less time pressure on completing it.

Prioritise your time: do not allow yourself or others to waste it

The first step is to be clear about your goals in your work and home life, or leisure-time. Then you need to structure sufficient time around these priorities. When an activity arises over which you have a choice, match it against your goals. If it takes you further away from your goals, then refuse to take it on, but if it coincides with your goals, consider whether you have time to fit it in.

Make sure that you spend your quality time doing the most important or complex jobs. It is all too easy to focus on getting small unimportant tasks done and to put off tackling the large ones, which then hang over you and make you feel guilty for leaving them unattended.

A high-priority task has to be done, a medium-priority job may be delegated, and a low-priority task should only be done if you have no medium- or high-priority tasks waiting, or if you are too jaded to tackle them.

The majority of your time should be devoted to pursuing your most important goals, and a small proportion of your time should be spent on less important matters.

Control interruptions

Interruptions are one of the biggest time-wasters, especially if someone else could have handled the problem or taken the message, or if no action was required. Even if an interruption is necessary, it may occur at the wrong time, wrecking your concentration or train of thought. Agree rules in your work-place with regard to who may be interrupted and when.

Include sufficient time for thinking, doing, meeting, developing and learning

You need to be fresh and creative in order to stay on top of the demands that are made on you. You can only manage this in the longer term if you have the right mix of stimulating work, personal and professional development and networking regularly timetabled into your daily schedule.

You will achieve more in designated sessions of quiet uninterrupted periods than in a longer period of time broken up by various activities. You need uninterrupted time for concentrating on planning, writing reports or analysing progress.

Try to set aside at least 10% of your time for dealing with unexpected tasks. In the unlikely event that everything goes smoothly and you do not need the extra time, it will be a bonus to have that additional space in which to catch up on the backlog of paperwork, or simply to spend a little more time talking to people about how they are feeling or what they are doing.

Delegate whatever and however you can

Only accept delegated work if you have the necessary skills, time and experience to do so.

If you are in a position to delegate work and responsibilities, decide what only *you* can do, and then delegate as much as possible of the rest to others. If you are more usually on the receiving end of delegated work, try to make sure that you understand what is required, and that you have the time, skills and experience necessary before agreeing or acquiescing to taking on the new work. If you do not have the time or skills for the additional work, negotiate in your most assertive manner how you will get the training and when you will do the work.

Do not consider delegation just at work, but also at home (cleaning, gardening, help from all of the family, etc.).

Control your work flow

Concentrate on one task at a time. Complete it and either move on to another job or take a short break to refresh yourself and clear your mind ready to start again. Do not move from one task to another or you will waste effort, as you will have to start thinking about the topic all over again each time you take it up.

You are likely to be more efficient if you group small similar tasks together, such as returning phone calls. Always have one or two small jobs put by or carried with you, so that if you are kept waiting you can get on with them and not waste time. Maintain control of your paperwork, and do not let it build up so that you feel overwhelmed, or you will put off tackling it altogether, or work more slowly because the enormity of the task depresses you.

Limit the time that you spend on the telephone. If you measure how long you talk for the next few times you are on the phone, you will probably be surprised by how many minutes the calls last for.

Minimise paperwork

Only pick up a piece of paper once, only start a job when you have time to finish it, deal with the most complicated task first whilst you are fresh, and delegate appropriately as far as possible.

Sort paperwork into the following categories:

- must be done today
- can wait a few days
- can wait a few weeks
- for someone else to do.

Much of the material in this section is derived from Chambers R (1999) *Survival Skills for GPs*. Radcliffe Medical Press, Oxford.

Games, activities and learning techniques

Exercise 14.1 Keep a log of daily activities

Why you should do this

To give people insight into how they spend their time, so that they can review whether they wish to change the balance of time that is spent on their various activities.

When to do this

In any workshop, or as homework, where participants are reviewing their time management.

What to do

Photocopy the daily log on page 144. Participants should record all of their activities each day for a week, including an off-duty period if possible. They should then sort the activities into three separate columns as follows:

- *personal needs*, including shopping, sleeping, domestic chores, bodily needs, etc.
- *work*, including reading work-related books, reports and papers
- *leisure*, including sport, relaxation, reading, music, etc.

Once they have worked out totals for the types of activities for each day, they should group the activities within the personal needs, work and leisure categories.

They should then compare several days of their daily recordings for these categories with the recommendations of the Health Education Authority (now the Health Development Agency) for a healthy lifestyle, which are as follows:

- 45–55% on personal needs
- 25–30% on work
- 20–25% on leisure.

How it works (insight)

Participants can look for any trends or patterns of activities (e.g. staying late at work or catching up on paperwork at home) from their daily activity logs. Comparing with their peers and with recommended guidelines will help participants to realise that the way in which they divide their own time may be abnormal, and may thus stimulate change.

Whom to engage

Anyone and everyone will benefit from reviewing the extent to which they achieve a good balance in the way in which they allocate time to essential, desirable and unimportant activities in their lives.

How much time you should allow

It should take up to 10 minutes each day to complete the log of time spent on various activities and to total the time within the three categories. Therefore a week of recording should take about an hour. The discussion in the workshop, comparison with peers and the guidelines might take up to an hour if participants start to map out changes to their usual routines.

What the facilitator should do

Stress the importance of the exercise if the participants are complaining about excessive demands at work, are facing new demands, or need to achieve a better balance between their work and home lives.

What to do next

Encourage participants to reflect on their own time logs after the workshop and discuss them with their partner or family at home, or with a work colleague. Encourage them to recruit others to help them to make sensible changes to their weekly schedules.

What makes it work better

A trusting atmosphere so that participants can share sensitive information about their feelings and frustrations.

What can go wrong

- Some of the participants may mock an individual's lack of balance (e.g. that they have spent no time on leisure activities).
- Participants may breech agreed rules about confidentiality and tell others outside the group the details of an individual's private life.

Exercise 14.2 Reduce time pressures at work

Why you should use this

To enable individuals to learn to plan to stay in control of their workload.

When to use this

In a workshop or as homework.

What to do

Participants look at the suggestions for reducing time pressures that are listed in Table 14.1 from the perspectives of an individual and an organisation.

DAILY LOG OF ACTIVITIES

TIME SPENT (TO NEAREST QUARTER OF AN HOUR) ON:					
Personal needs (shopping, washing, domestic chores, sleeping)		*Work*		*Leisure*	
Activity	*Time spent*	*Activity*	*Time spent*	*Activity*	*Time spent*
	Total/day:		Total/day:		Total/day:

Table 14.1:   Suggestions for reducing time pressures

What you can do as an individual	*What the organisation can do*
Plan well in advance to avoid crises	Plan well in advance to avoid crises
Set aside 10% of your time for unexpected tasks	Organise time management training for staff
Do not book a meeting too close to a previous commitment which may over-run	Match staff numbers to volume of work
Build in time for reflection and planning	Organise realistic work plans
Minimise interruptions	Discourage social chit-chat in work time
Make maximum use of technology	Make maximum use of technology
Other:	Other:

They should add any other ideas that they have to both lists. They should then work in pairs or small groups to draw up action plans for up to five specific ways of reducing time pressures in their work setting – what they can do themselves and what the organisation can do.

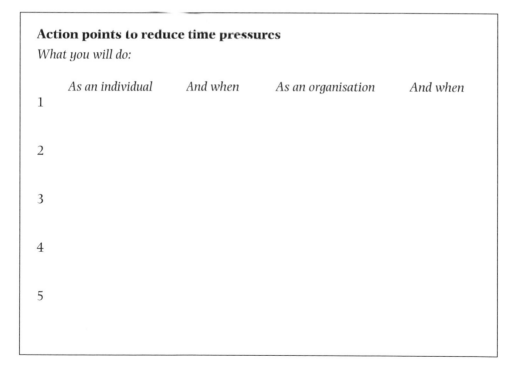

How it works (insight)

This exercise forces participants to realise the varied solutions that there are for reducing time pressures, and that they are not helpless. It also helps them to understand that they cannot reduce time pressures as individuals in isolation from the rest of the organisation. Both the individual and the organisation need to work together to reduce time pressures effectively.

Whom to engage

Managers and staff – anyone and everyone.

How much time you should allow

Encourage brainstorming and discussion by allowing about 90 minutes for the exercise.

What the facilitator should do

When describing the exercise, have plenty of illustrative examples of actions that have worked elsewhere when people have tackled time pressures as individuals or organisations. Intervene if participants wander away from the task by talking about the negative effects of time pressures rather than making positive plans to tackle such pressures.

What to do next

Try to arrange some type of follow-up review of intended action, perhaps as pairs of participants or as a working party at organisational level.

What makes it work better

- A mixed group of staff from different disciplines, managers and clinicians will enhance the understanding of both individual and organisational perspectives and hopefully improve the subsequent action plans.
- An external person or new member of staff might feed in their relatively independent views of the time pressures that they perceive and the degree of effort that individuals and the organisation currently seem to be putting into reducing such pressures.

What can go wrong

It is all very well to make resolutions, but quite another matter to put those resolutions into practice.

Exercise 14.3 Rushing through an activity often does not save time in the long run

Why you should use this

To demonstrate that doing things too quickly can be counter-productive if you make mistakes or omissions. 'More haste, less speed', as they say.

When to use this

When working with a group of at least six people who are learning about time management.

What to do

Show the following text to the participants for 45 seconds. Make sure that everyone has an equal opportunity to read the text for the same amount of time. Ask those present to count the number of occurrences of the letter 'f' in the following text while remaining silent. Then invite people to indicate their answer by raising their hands when you as the facilitator state the number of occurrences of the letter 'f' that they may have counted in the paragraph. Call out ascending numbers, starting from a low number such as 6, 7, 8, etc., and working upwards.

> The sheriff forgot his badge when he went to the saloon. Five men were fighting on the floor of the veranda. If he handcuffed the first man of the five, he thought that he would stop the fighting.

How it works (insight)

Participants will scan the text quickly because of the time pressure that you as facilitator impose on them. Many will tend to have ignored the small words and merely counted the number of 'f's in the more important words, such as the nouns and verbs.

Whom to engage

This exercise works with anyone, but especially professionals who are used to operating quickly.

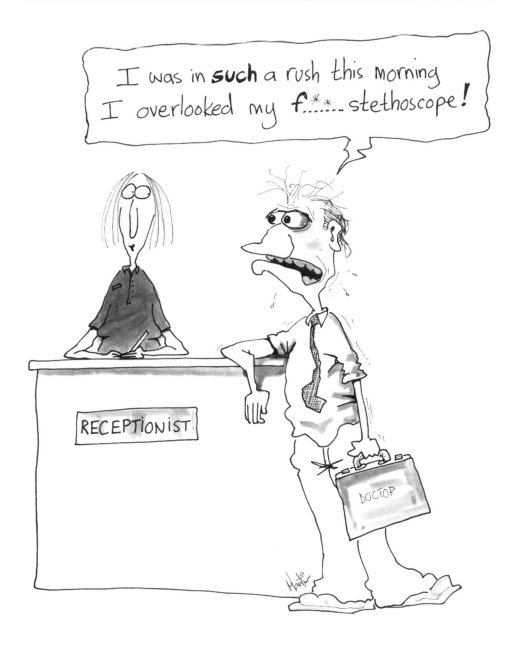

How much time you should allow

Allow about 5 minutes to give the instructions to count the number of occurrences of the letter 'f', 45 seconds to read the text, and a few minutes to elicit participants' answers and debrief.

What the facilitator should do

Make sure that everyone has an equal opportunity to read the text. Set the scene so that everyone is concentrating and is prepared to start the exercise together. Urge everyone to remain silent and keep their answer to themselves until they are invited to indicate their tally. Give the true answer (14 in our example exercise here) and explain the purpose of the exercise and why others will have omitted to notice some letter 'f's.

What to do next

You need do little else, as the realisation of how easy it was to miss the 'f's in such a short paragraph should have made an impact on the individuals participating in the exercise.

What makes it work better

- You can make up your own paragraph that is relevant to the discipline or work done by the participants.
- Keep the word count relatively low (e.g. less than 40 words) and make sure that several small linking words are included if you compose your own text.
- Choose a different letter, such as 'n', which also has several two-letter word alternatives such as 'in', 'on' and 'an'.

What can go wrong

- Even if people have done this exercise before and know that they must be careful to count the 'f's from each word systematically, they will still have difficulty in recognising each 'f' when working at speed – so it is difficult to go wrong.
- The facilitator might spoil the surprise impact of the exercise on 'first-timers' by explaining the likely variation of the group's response prior to conducting the exercise.

15

Stress management and support

What is stress?

Stress is very difficult to define, as it is such a vague word and everyone interprets it differently. Stress is equivalent to a person's perception of the pressure upon them, or the 'three-way relationship between demands on a person, that person's feelings about those demands and their ability to cope with those demands'.[1] In other words, a particular event or task can be very stressful for you on one day but not on another, depending on how you are feeling and what other pressures are being exerted on you.

In general, stress occurs in situations where the workload is high, control over the workload is limited, and too little support or help is available. Many people would say that they know when they are feeling stressed even if they cannot specify exactly what stress is!

Is stress bad for you?

The answer to this question depends on how much stress you are under, for how long it is applied, whether you feel powerless to stand up to the stress, or whether you can overcome it. A moderate amount of stress is necessary to perform well at work and to maintain a zest for life. Zero stress may lead to boredom, whereas too much stress over too long a period will render you indecisive, exhausted or 'burnt out'.

Stress affects the whole of today's society – no professional group is unique in reporting escalating levels of stress and low morale. In a typical week, one million of the 24 million people in the UK's workforce took one day off work, and up to 40% of absenteeism is thought to be due to mental or emotional problems. In the health setting, caring for others creates additional stresses due to daily exposure to human distress and ill health, and the daily striving for perfection in relieving all suffering and never making mistakes.[2]

Is stress an integral part of the job?

It is important to distinguish between an occasional event or task that creates the highest levels of stress, and those that account for the most frequent reports of stress. For example, an official complaint against you might cause terrific levels of stress, but hopefully rarely happens, whereas minor hassles at work may be a frequent cause of stress. A steady relentless dripping of stress-provoking situations may be just as likely to create a stressed worker as a crisis event with monumental stress attached to it.

Stress at work does not happen 'in a vacuum'. Pressures and problems at home often overflow into how someone feels and performs at work, and the effects of stress at work are often taken home and unfairly dumped there. Different people experience various proportions and mixes of physical, mental, emotional and behavioural symptoms. Significant life events may be the real cause of stress being experienced at work.

There are three types of responses to stress, namely physiological, psychological and behavioural reactions. The ways in which we respond depend on personal factors such as age, gender, personality, and previous family and personal experiences, as well as coping ability and other organisational options.

Stress management

The types of practical methods that people can use to cope with stress at work include the following:

* seeking support from colleagues
* sharing problems with colleagues
* adopting better time management practices
* more appropriate booking times for appointments and meetings
* increased protected time off duty, limiting working hours to those for which one is contracted
* admitting doubts and worries to others
* achieving a better balance between work and home commitments.

Avoiding the seven deadly sins of the workaholic is another good starting point for increased well-being and stress management.

1   Stop being a perfectionist.
2   Do not judge your mistakes too harshly.
3   Resist the desire to control everything.
4   Learn to decline extra commitments assertively if you are already pressed for time.
5   Look after your personal health and fitness.

6   Allow time for personal growth, the family and leisure.
7   Do not be too proud to ask for help.

To stay on top, you may need to regain your enthusiasm for learning and your quest for knowledge and understanding. The personal satisfaction derived from completing a project, degree course or some other educational experience is likely to make any professional feel more fulfilled, and to reawaken an interest in all aspects of work.

It is not stress itself that is the damaging factor, but your inability to cope with it. In a changing world, people need to learn new ways of coping, as that way lies survival.

Being assertive

Assertiveness is about knowing and practising your rights – to change your mind, make mistakes, refuse demands, express emotions, be yourself without having to act for other people's benefit, and make decisions or statements without always having to justify them.

It takes practice to be assertive   so get some practice in at work and at home. The greatest challenge may be being assertive with yourself so that you do not agree to take on additional tasks that are not essential for you to undertake, or that fall outside your own priority areas.

How often do you hear people saying 'No, no ... no ... oh ... alright then, I suppose so'? Listen carefully to what is being asked of you, weigh up the time, effort and skills that the task or activity will take, and the extent to which it is an essential, desirable or possible feature of your working or home life – and decide on your assertive response.

The chief points to remember about being assertive are listed below.

1   Say 'No' clearly and then move away or change the subject. Keep repeating 'No' – do not allow yourself to be diverted.
2   Be honest and direct with everyone.
3   Do not apologise or justify yourself more than is reasonable.
4   Offer a workable compromise and negotiate an agreement that suits you and the other party.
5   Pause before answering a 'Yes' that you will regret. Delay your response and give yourself more time to think by asking for more information.
6   Be aware of your body language and keep it as assertive as possible. Match your tone to your words (do not smile if you are giving a serious message).
7   Use the 'broken-record' technique – persistently repeat your message in a calm manner to someone who is trying to pressurise you. Do not allow yourself to be side-tracked.

8   Show that you are listening to the other person's point of view and
     giving them a fair hearing.
9   Practise expressing your opinion and rights rather than expecting other
     people to guess what you want.
10   Do not be too hard on yourself if you make a mistake – everyone is
     human.
11   Be confident enough to change your mind if that is appropriate.
12   It can be assertive to say nothing at all.

Support

Research into stress has shown that people with the best social supports,
who interact well with other people, are able to cope with stress and are least
affected by it.

Be prepared to ask for help. This is not a sign of weakness or ignorance.
Support networks may be used for another professional opinion or for emotional assistance. Support for colleagues should be non-judgemental, and a
culture should be developed at work in which people do not feel embarrassed
or 'silly' because they are asking for help.

A close and supportive partner and family at home can be a good safe
place to offload and share worries about work, so long as this does not stress
relationships unduly.

Much of the material in this chapter is derived from Chambers R (1999)
Survival Skills for GPs. Radcliffe Medical Press, Oxford.

References

1   Richards C (1989) *The Health of Doctors.* King's Fund, London.
2   Chambers R (1999) *Survival Skills for GPs.* Radcliffe Medical Press, Oxford.

Games, activities and learning techniques

Exercise 15.1 Draw up a personal map of support mechanisms in your life

Why you should do this

To realise for yourself the components of your life that lend you support and
that you can build upon.

When to use this

With a group of people who have been meeting regularly and who feel comfortable about sharing feelings. Alternatively, you can use it on a one-to-one basis.

What to do

- *Stage 1*: Draw yourself in the middle of a piece of plain paper. Then draw pictures to represent all of the sources of support in your life – people, things, situations, environment, etc. Link each picture to you in the centre with a line (*see* the example in Figure 15.1).
- *Stage 2*: Next add drawings of the other sources of support that you have used in the past but not employed for a while, and add other pictures of the extra sources of support you would like to have. Link each picture to you in the centre of the page.
- *Stage 3*: Draw in the barriers that prevent you from using these sources of support across the line linking that particular source with you.
- *Stage 4*: Share and compare your personal support map with someone else who has drawn one. Discuss which are your strongest sources of support, which are the ones you would like to enhance, the barriers that prevent you from making more of your sources of support, and what is missing.

How it works (insight)

This exercise helps people to acknowledge and review the extent and type of the sources of support that exist for them at work and outside work. The exercise may give participants insight into how sources of support have withered away, or how they are taking partners, etc., for granted and not devoting enough quality time to their supporters. It may enable them to define the balance between work and home that they need to regain in their life. It might help individuals to recognise the barriers that prevent them from spending time and effort on leisure activities or maintaining relationships.

Whom to engage

This exercise works for anyone and everyone who wants to review and maintain or build up support mechanisms.

How much time you should allow

Allow 20 to 30 minutes for stages 1, 2 and 3, and a further 20 minutes for stage 4.

What the facilitator should do

Keep the exercise moving, giving out instructions for the progressive stages 1, 2 and 3. Discourage participants from intense or emotional discussion at stage 4 if the exercise is being undertaken in a group setting as a preliminary activity to other educational activities.

What to do next

Encourage the participants to make a plan to remove at least one barrier in order to enhance at least one source of support.

What makes it work better

An atmosphere of trust and mutual respect both between the participants and between the participants and the facilitator.

What can go wrong

One or more individuals may become distressed if the exercise strikes home and they suddenly realise the lack of sources of support in their lives.

Exercise 15.2 Consequences: understanding the consequences of stress at work

Why you should use this

To free participants to be able to talk about sensitive subjects such as stress (its causes, effects and solutions) without the material being attributable to individuals.

To help participants to understand that everyone is subject to stress, and to be more aware of the different sources of stress. To learn about various stress-coping mechanisms that work for other people.

When to use this

If you wish to encourage a group of people to engage in open discussion and exchange of tips and techniques about sensitive topics such as feelings, beliefs, money, sex, etc.

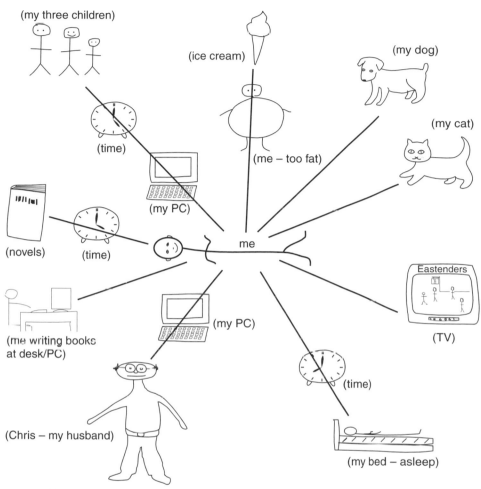

(my three children)

(ice cream)

(my dog)

(time)

(me – too fat)

(my cat)

(my PC)

(novels)   (time)   me

Eastenders

(me writing books
at desk/PC)   (my PC)   (TV)

(time)

(Chris – my husband)

(my bed – asleep)

Key: see instructions in exercise.
The various people and objects giving support are arranged around
the person in the centre, linked by straight lines. If anything obstructs
the supportive source, this is drawn across the relevant line.

Figure 15.1:   Example of a personal support map.

What to do

This exercise is adapted from the childhood game of 'Consequences'.
Participants should sit in a circle.

1   Each participant writes down a key stress related to work for them – as
    word, phrase or short sentence (statement 1). Each person should fold the
    paper over so that statement 1 is obscured, and should pass the paper on
    to the person on their right-hand side and receive a similar piece of paper
    from the person sitting on their left-hand side.

2   Each participant now writes down a few words or a short sentence about
     what physical effects significant stress has on them (e.g. racing heart,
     headaches, etc.). This is statement 2. As before, each participant should
     fold the paper over so that the person next in line to receive it cannot
     read statements 1 or 2, and again each should pass the paper with
     completed statements 1 and 2 to the person on their right-hand side.
3   Continue with the same procedure for five more statements about the
     following:
     •   the mental effects that significant stress has on them (e.g. poor
          concentration)
     •   the effects that significant stress has on their behaviour (e.g. over-
          eating, excessive drinking, arriving late for work)
     •   the effects that significant stress has on their relationships with other
          people at work
     •   their favoured solutions for stress at work (up to three)
     •   how they will know that they have controlled stress at work.

The facilitator should then collect all of the papers and read out the 'consequences' of stress and the suggested solutions.

The participants should now discuss whether the solutions on the individual answer-sheets are appropriate to the preceding information about the
nature of the stress and its effects, and if not, what would be suitable coping
mechanisms.

How it works (insight)

The exercise should enable the participants to realise that (almost) everyone
else suffers from stress at work, and to be more aware of the different sources
of stress in the workplace. The way in which the exercise is arranged means
that no one should be able to work out who wrote down what, and participants can be more honest and open than they would be if they had had to say
what stress they personally experienced and how it made them feel. They should
learn how others cope with stress and gain some new ideas for themselves.

Whom to engage

Everyone has the potential to suffer from stress. Any stress management
workshop could use this exercise, or any educational group of professionals
that wants to prevent or reduce stress at work, as it interferes with performance and ability to learn.

The minimum number of participants for diversity and anonymity is
probably six. There is no maximum number for the first stage of compiling
the 'consequences' lists of stressors, effects and solutions. A large number

of participants can then break down into small groups of no more than 12 people to allow discussion.

How much time you should allow

Allow at least one hour. The exercise itself takes 15 minutes, but discussing the range of responses line by line takes a considerable amount of time. The exact time will depend on the number of participants and the range of their responses, as well as the extent of discussion about the appropriateness of coping methods for the stresses that someone else wrote down.

What the facilitator should do

Explain the exercise carefully, as the activity may seem pointless to participants at first as they continually fill in each new statement and pass the papers on, anticipating that the resulting answer-sheets may be nonsensical. Thus the facilitator needs to urge their co-operation and persuade them to have faith in the potential benefits of the exercise.

What to do next

As they discuss the links between stressors, their effects and appropriate solutions, participants should be formulating their own mental action plans to minimise stress in their own lives. This should lead to personal action plans or organisational/workplace stress management programmes, or both.

What makes it work better

Pre prepared sheets with instructions, space for the answers to be filled in, and dotted lines indicating where the paper should be folded (*see* page 160 for an example). The participants may swap partly completed answer-sheets across the circle at interim stages in the exercise, to increase the likelihood of anonymity.

What can go wrong

- People recognising other individuals' handwriting and identifying who wrote what.
- One or two participants refusing to join in and pass their paper on, so disrupting the circulation of answer-sheets to neighbouring participants.
- One or two participants misunderstanding the instructions and writing their answers in the wrong place on both sides of the paper so that the resulting answer-sheet has gaps in the pathway from causes to effects to solutions.

Example of 'Consequences' response sheet. **Fold top of page down to here.**

1   Fold here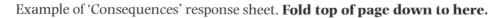
Write down a *key stress related to work* for you as a word, a phrase or a short sentence (not an essay!).

Before you pass this paper on to the person sitting on your right-hand side and receive a similar piece of paper from the person sitting on your left-hand side, fold the paper at the line above so that the statement you have just written is obscured.

2   Fold here ---
Write down a few words or a short sentence about the *physical effects* that significant stress has on you (e.g. racing heart, headaches, etc.).

Then fold over the paper at 2 above so that the person on your right-hand side cannot read what you have written. Pass this paper to the person sitting on your right-hand side and receive a similar paper from the person on your left-hand side.

3   Fold here ---
Write down a few words or a short sentence about the *mental effects* that significant stress has on you (e.g. poor concentration, etc.).

Then fold over the paper at 3 above so that the person on your right-hand side cannot read what you have written. Pass this paper to your neighbour on your right-hand side.

4   Fold here ---
Write down a few words or a short sentence about the effects that significant stress has on *your behaviour* (e.g. over-eating, excessive alcohol consumption, etc.).

Then fold over the paper at 4 above so that the person on your right-hand side cannot read what you have written. Pass this paper to your neighbour on your right-hand side.

Fold top of page down to here.

5   Fold here --
Write down a few words or a short sentence about the effects that significant stress has on *your relationships with other people at work* (e.g. rows, misunder-standings, etc.).

Then fold over the paper at 5 above so that the person on your right-hand side cannot read what you have written. Pass this paper to your neighbour on your right-hand side.

6   Fold here --
Briefly describe *your favoured solutions* (up to three) for combating significant stress at work that usually work for you.

Then fold over the paper at 6 above so that the person on your right-hand side cannot read what you have written. Pass this paper to your neighbour on your right-hand side.

7   Fold here --
Briefly describe *how you will know that you have controlled stress at work.*

Then fold over the paper at 7 above so that the person on your right-hand side cannot read what you have written. Pass this paper to the facilitator.

16

Multidisciplinary learning

Multidisciplinary learning (e.g. between those working in health and non-health organisations) is still uncommon. This type of learning is about organising everyone's part in learning so that individuals in the team are competent to deliver the care and services that you have planned. This will involve individuals in the team and from different workplaces learning together or separately, in-house or on external courses in whatever way is most effective for addressing their learning needs and anticipated roles and responsibilities.

Multidisciplinary and multiprofessional learning does not mean that everyone learns the same as everyone else at the same time. There will always be a place for uniprofessional education. Some clinical or organisational subjects are so specialised that they only apply to one particular discipline or subspecialty of doctors, nurses, therapists or managers. There will be situations where participants from one discipline are not sufficiently confident to be comfortable about being taught alongside other learners from a traditionally dominant discipline, such as doctors. Sometimes the learning needs of one professional will be more basic than those of the rest of the team or from other disciplines, where individuals have varying expertise.

It is important that you clearly identify where team or multiprofessional learning offers the best solution, and take full advantage of learning on the job – on the ward, or in the clinic or surgery.

The effect of tribalism on multiprofessional learning

The traditional models of training of many professional groups produce a strong sense of professional identity which is reinforced by postgraduate study and examinations. This strong identity is seen in the training of doctors, but is also prevalent in the training of nurses, midwives, occupational therapists, physiotherapists, etc. The pain and struggle of the training programmes, the secondary socialisation and the initiation into the professional subgroup (e.g. a surgeon or intensive-care-unit nurse) echo other rites of passage or initiation rites of primitive tribes. It is therefore not surprising that members of a profession develop a strong tribal identity. People will often fight to defend their exclusive membership of their professional group or 'tribe' even in the face of overwhelming evidence that working (and learning) with members of other 'tribes' will produce benefits for all. You may think that this is a strong analogy, but just consider the opposition that many general practitioners have presented to the introduction of nurse prescribing in primary care.

Loss of professional identity is similar to bereavement. The symptoms can include numbness, denial, yearning, depression, guilt and aggression. Therefore it is important that a teacher or facilitator remembers that some of the reasons for the failure of multiprofessional education may be the result of powerful emotions akin to the loss of a loved one – in this case the threat to the professional identity of the learner.

Counselling is effective in dealing with bereavement and grief in the relatives of patients. Similarly, educational counselling may be needed if the development of a multiprofessional learning session or course is being blocked by an individual or professional group. One-to-one counselling should help those concerned to come to terms with the (potential) loss of identity and allow them to reflect on their concerns. Involving the individual(s) in the planning of future learning activities is also helpful.

Multiprofessional small-group learning will help the team to develop if the subjects of the learning are relevant to all participants. It is useful to spend time sharing thoughts, problem solving and reflecting. Shared reflective learning will help to overcome exclusion and encourage true partnerships to develop.

Multidisciplinary learning will enable individuals in that team to develop:

- new roles
- respect for other professions and colleagues
- an atmosphere of openness and trust
- real communication between colleagues
- an appreciation of the strengths of the diversity of other professionals and the complex nature of professional judgement and ways of working
- a common set of values and attitudes
- an understanding of the contribution that other professionals can make and how different professions work together best
- ways to overcome the isolation of various professionals, especially those who usually work alone
- a more appropriate skill mix of healthcare professionals to deliver particular services.

This approach to learning is at the heart of personal, professional, work-based or organisational learning plans. It is impossible for an individual who is working alone to identify their own learning needs reliably, or to plan their learning in a cost-effective or systematic manner so that it fits with the overall workplace plan and patients' needs. This team-based consultation about individuals' learning needs identified by annual appraisals and discussion and the ensuing collaboration over the team's learning plan is all part of multidisciplinary learning.

Further reading

There are many relevant articles in the *Journal of Interprofessional Care*.

Chambers R and Wall D (2000) *Teaching Made Easy*. Radcliffe Medical Press, Oxford.

National Health Service Executive (1998) *Working Together. Securing a quality workforce for the NHS*. Department of Health, London.

Standing Committee on Postgraduate Medical and Dental Education (SCOPME) (1997) *Multiprofessional Working and Learning: sharing the educational challenge*. SCOPME, London.

Standing Committee on Postgraduate Medical and Dental Education (SCOPME) (1998) *Continuing Professional Development for Doctors and Dentists*. SCOPME, London.

Games, activities and learning techniques

Exercise 16.1 Multidisciplinary learning from a spoof exercise

Why you should do this

To increase people's awareness of the varied skill mix within the team and enable them to appreciate the knowledge and skills of other team members.

When to use this

In a situation where some participants in the group have differing baseline knowledge and skills to others. The exercise will help all group members to reach a common understanding about a topic, where those with more expert knowledge and skills automatically share these with 'novices' or those from different disciplines.

What to do

Prepare a 'spoof' report of an activity that is relevant to the theme of the learning objectives of the event. An example is given on page 167. Ask the group to brainstorm on what mistakes and omissions occur in the spoof report. You might start by inviting general comments, and then ask the group to identify specific mistakes or omissions against a checklist of important aspects.

Finally, review best practice in this area, which will be the alternative version of the 'spoof' report that contained the mistakes and omissions.

How it works (insight)

The exercise really holds people's interest as they spot mistakes with child-like glee. Spotting the gaps is more difficult, and will lead to a discussion among the team members as some identify gaps of which others are unaware. Thus the team members teach each other and come to an agreement about best practice with regard to the roles and responsibilities of all the team.

Whom to engage

Any group – for example, a multidisciplinary group meeting as in the example given here.

How much time you should allow

Spotting the mistakes is a short exercise for which you should allow, say, 15 minutes. Recognising the gaps and discussing them and their importance will take longer and depend on the topic – say another 45 minutes for the example given here.

What the facilitator should do

Encourage those participants with more expert knowledge and skills to hold back and let those who are 'novices' spot the mistakes first. Then encourage everyone to contribute and ask the experts on particular features of the exercise to explain why there are gaps that should be rectified, not merely to point out the omissions.

What to do next

Encourage the multidisciplinary group to devise a policy that incorporates risk management to ensure that the mistakes which occurred in the spoof exercise do not occur in real life.

What makes it work better

There should be some obvious mistakes that everyone can spot, some humorous ones to lighten the mood of the participants, and some can be more subtle for experts on the topic – so that there is something for everyone.

What can go wrong

The exercise may be pitched incorrectly so that the participants do not recognise the mistakes and omissions in the 'spoof' report and they think that the text is correct.

Example of a 'spoof' report that you could use for a multidisciplinary learning exercise

Producing a newsletter for patients

Peter, the practice manager of the Ever-ready practice in Brightown, decided to produce a fortnightly newsletter for patients. He wanted the sort of people who rarely came to see a doctor to attend the new screening clinics they were setting up in the practice for chlamydia, testicular cancer and obesity. Peter knew that the GPs would agree so long as he produced the newsletter at no cost to the practice. For the first issue, he commissioned his wife, who was a slimming club organiser, to write a couple of articles on losing weight. He had some good leaflets in a drawer on checking for testicular cancer that included some shock statistics, and the practice secretary typed these up for him. The practice nurse had her arm twisted for the article about the frequency of chlamydia and the association with infertility. Peter was able to describe all of the new services – they had managed to fit them all in with little disruption to the practice, between morning and evening surgery, without altering the surgery hours. When the first issue of the newsletter was complete, he had 400 copies printed and put them out on display in the waiting-room. They all went in the first week – a great success and at no cost. His wife's slimming club organisation had paid for the printing in return for a front-page advert.

So what are the mistakes?

Too numerous to mention here ... and if we (the authors) do not spot them all, you might judge us harshly!

Some of the mistakes that might be mentioned in the discussion would include the following:

- the lack of consultation with the GPs and the practice team about the venture
- the siting of such screening services in an afternoon, which may not be appropriate for the 'client' group

- the lack of consultation with the patient groups – do they want a news-letter or the new services, especially the target groups of young people and those who are obese?
- the provision of newsletters to those using the service and not to non-users, which had been one of the original goals
- the lack of ownership of the team in contributing articles
- the inappropriate authorship of the articles – biased, out of date, reluctant non-expert
- staff time must be costed and not assumed to be 'free'
- the advert for the slimming clinic might not be consistent with ethical guidelines for advertising
- the article and advert from the slimming-club perspective might conflict with the weight management approach promoted in the new 'obesity screening' service (e.g. it might not promote increasing physical activity or the use of drugs to the same extent as the practice approach)
- a fortnightly newsletter from a practice would be costly and exacting.

And so on.

Some of the gaps that might be mentioned include the following:

- lack of prior networking with the genitourinary clinic service – close working would be required for contact tracing with chlamydia
- lack of prior networking with the local health promotion service who might help to provide up-to-date advice on detecting testicular cancer and preventing obesity
- setting a budget for the enterprise
- the creation of a newsletter as an ad hoc initiative without it being part of a co-ordinated strategy for improving communication with all subgroups within the patient population.

And so on.

In summary, this 'spoof' report is given as an example of how the exercise can lead on to discussion of the detailed planning and organisation that are necessary before any new service is set up. All members of a multidisciplinary team should be able to contribute to the example of this exercise, which includes organisational and clinical elements, the patients' and staff's perspectives, policy, planning and provision.

Exercise 16.2 Workshops without any curriculum

This exercise is sometimes known as the 'Oslo' way because a well-publicised medical education seminar that adopted this format was held in that city in the 1990s.

Why you should do this

Having no pre-set curriculum enables the participants to set their current learning objectives for the event.

When to use this

An arrangement such as this exercise will be suitable for a topic where there is more than one way forward, with many diverse factors to consider, where people would like to share their experiences and ideas and do not want to be limited by preconceptions or a planned programme.

What to do

1 Invite potential participants to a seminar with a theme but without a programme. Be explicit that participants will have to work hard and bring to the group the issues and challenges that they want to debate.
2 Each participant should prepare material for a possible workshop or session in which they hope to interest others.
3 Would-be workshop leaders briefly describe the workshop that they hope to run by placing a notice on a noticeboard the evening before a morning session, before lunch for an afternoon session, etc.
4 Those who wish to attend such a workshop sign up, and the organisers find them a room. Any very similar workshops are combined by agreement.
5 Participants get together as a group once or twice a day.

How it works (insight)

Participants can develop the theme and the ideas in the direction in which they wish to progress with little constraint. New leaders with different expertise take over as the direction meanders or deviates from the initial workshop.

Whom to engage

This exercise could attract the type of people who usually lead others (e.g. representatives who lead a primary care organisation), or it could be used in a multidisciplinary general practice team.

How much time you should allow

Allow as much time as is available – there is no end to the exercise to define the time spent, as participants can just keep on going and developing the theme. The exercise is time limited by the extent to which participants can be released from their everyday work. Realistically, such an unstructured session might extend from a half day to several days.

What the facilitator should do

Make sure that there are enough meeting rooms to house all of the workshops. Provide any materials that the workshop leaders may require (audiovisual equipment, etc.). Try to discourage one or two individuals from dominating the proceedings – everyone needs an equal opportunity to develop their own and others' ideas. Be flexible!

What to do next

Make sure that the learning event is not so unstructured that it becomes a talking shop and too little is achieved that can be implemented afterwards.

What makes it work better

Commitment from people who can 'make things happen' after the event.

What can go wrong

The 'wrong' people may attend, who are unwilling to throw themselves into this developmental opportunity and would prefer a more traditional structured event in which they can take a more passive role.

17

Evaluation

Evaluation is an essential component of any programme or service – plan it in advance and incorporate it in any plan from the beginning. Time and effort spent on evaluation should be in proportion to the activity that is being evaluated. Keep it as simple as possible – do not waste resources on unnecessarily bureaucratic evaluation.

Design the evaluation so that you:

- specify the event (e.g. a service) to be evaluated – define broad issues, set priorities against strategic goals, time and resources, seek agreement on the nature and scope of the task
- describe the expected impact of the programme or activity and who will be affected by it
- define the criteria for success – these might relate to structure, process or outcome
- identify the information/evidence required to demonstrate the achievements of the programme or activity. These sources of evidence might include observing behaviour, data from existing records and prospective recording by the subjects of the programme or by the recipients and staff of the activity
- determine the time-frame
- determine who will collect the data for all stages of the delivery of the programme or activity, and the respective deadlines
- review and refine the objectives of the programme or activity, and check that they are appropriate for the outcomes and impact you expect.

What to evaluate

There are many varied approaches to evaluation, some of which are listed below.

1   Adopt any or all of the six aspects of the health service's performance assessment framework, namely health improvement, fair access, effective delivery, efficiency, patient/carer experience, health outcomes.

2   Agree milestones and goals at specific stages in your programme, or adopt
    others (e.g. in the National Service Frameworks for coronary heart
    disease or mental health).

3   Evaluate the extent to which you achieve the outcome(s) starting with an
    objective, or you might evaluate how conducive the context of the pro-
    gramme or activity is to achieving the anticipated outcomes, or both. It
    may seem 'back to front' to set out the outcomes and then work backwards
    to first agreeing the context that will be needed and then the objective(s)
    that will achieve the outcome(s), but this is how the 'theory of change'
    works.[1]

4   Break down the project cycle into four stages:[2]
    • review of progress
    • agree the plan
    • implement the plan
    • demonstrate what you have achieved.
    Set goals or milestones as interim measures for all four of these stages,
    and evaluate the extent to which you complete the various aspects of the
    project as planned.

5   Undertake regular audits of aspects of the structure, process and outcome
    of a service or project to see whether you have achieved what you expected
    when you established the criteria and standards of the audit programme.

6   Evaluate the various components of a new system or programme (the
    activities, personnel involved, provision of services, organisational struc-
    ture, precise goals and interventions).

7   Measure success by how effective the team is[3] (*see* Chapter 7 on team-
    work), and evaluate whether the following are present:
    • clear team goals and objectives
    • accountability and authority
    • individual roles for members
    • shared tasks
    • regular internal formal and informal communication
    • full participation by members
    • confrontation of conflict
    • feedback to individuals
    • feedback on team performance
    • outside recognition of a team
    • two-way external communication
    • team rewards.

8   Evaluate the quality of service delivery by looking at people, environment
    and process (*see* Chapter 13 on organisational management).

9   Evaluate the aspects of care that are most highly valued by patients, namely:
    • availability and accessibility – appointments, waiting times, physical
      access and telephone access

- technical competence, including the knowledge, skills and effective-ness of the treatment provided by health professionals
- communication skills, including providing time, exploring patients' needs, listening, explaining, giving information and sharing decisions
- interpersonal attributes, including humaneness, caring attitude, sup-portiveness and trust
- organisation of care, including continuity of care, co-ordination of care and availability of on-site services.

References

1   Pawson R and Tilley N (2000) *Realistic Evaluation.* Sage, London.
2   Wood L (2001) *Review, Agree, Implement, Demonstrate.* National Clinical Govern-ance Support Team, Leicester.
3   Hart E and Fletcher J (1999) Learning how to change: a selective analysis of literature and experience of how teams learn and organisations change. *J Interprof Care.* **13**: 53–63.

Games, activities and learning techniques

Exercise 17.1 Three-months reminder: a self-evaluation

Why you should use this

To encourage your learners to make a pledge about what they will achieve as a result of the learning by a specified time (e.g. three months).

When to use this

On the last day of a course or any learning session in which participants have had an opportunity to make an action plan.

What to do

Give a blank postcard to each participant, and invite each of them to address the postcard back to themselves at their home or work address. They should add up to 40 words or so as a message to themselves that describes what they would like to have achieved within the specified period.

You should then collect the completed postcards and post them back to the participants at the agreed time.

How it works (insight)

Seeing the goal(s) set out in their own handwriting is a very powerful force. It immediately transports the participants back to the learning event when they had protected time to reflect on their work or home situation and the barriers to progress, and could think objectively about what needed to be done.

Whom to engage

Anyone attending a learning event, of any discipline or seniority. All participants should have one or more goals for the application of the new knowledge, skills or attitudes gained from attending the event.

How much time you should allow

Allow about five minutes to undertake the task.

What the facilitator should do

Encourage everyone to complete a postcard, and arrange this so that they are not overlooked by their neighbour and can make a personal resolution that will not be scorned by others. Gather up the cards and put them away so that they are not left lying around. Leave yourself, or the secretary who is assisting you, a reminder to post the cards on the right date (i.e. three months later).

What to do next

Participants who have not achieved their goal(s) by the specified time should consider why this is so, and either make a more realistic action plan or devise a new plan to overcome the barriers to change.

What makes it work better

- Have a choice of different postcards with a variety of pictures that make the exercise more fun as individuals select the card that they prefer. The postcards might be humorous, scenic or carry a message.
- Give the learners some advance notice of the exercise so that they can be formulating their message(s) to themselves in advance of completing the task.

What can go wrong

- Despite your best efforts, the participants may confer, thereby risking some individuals being ridiculed by others.
- When the postcard arrives at their home or work address, the participant may not be as happy about others reading their resolutions on an open postcard as they anticipated they would be while they were cocooned on the course.

Exercise 17.2 Take an IQ test

Why you should use this

To lighten the mood of the meeting by inserting a childlike task, but at the same time point out that the participants need to reflect on the tasks they are given and not simply react in the first way they think of.

When to use this

In a plenary group, perhaps after lunch or after a break to recapture the momentum of an earlier session. It could be set on general knowledge or on the topic of the learning event, in which case it could be used at any time in the educational session to provide a change of pace or style.

What to do

Prepare a list of general open questions or questions with a set of options of answers, or set the questions on the theme of the event. Include plenty of 'catch' questions where the correct answer is not the most obvious one that comes to mind (*see* page 177 for an example). Distribute a copy to each participant, and invite them to complete it under 'examination conditions' without conferring and within a specified time period.

Then give out the correct answers either as a copy for everyone or by means of the overhead projector. You could ask how many people gave correct answers by requesting a show of hands, starting from the highest possible number and working downwards.

How it works (insight)

The exercise is anonymous so that people can answer honestly. It brings people up with a jolt to realise they have been caught out – and they can extrapolate from that learning to their everyday life, where they realise that they should reflect and think laterally before jumping to the first solution that occurs to them.

Whom to engage

This exercise is suitable for anyone and everyone, depending on the pitch and level of the questions.

How much time you should allow

Allow less than 5 minutes if there are 10 or fewer questions which are reasonably simple. The idea is for people to respond from their 'gut' feelings rather than spending time pondering before answering.

What the facilitator should do

Find some questions. Borrow those in our example or make up others with similar 'catches'.

What to do next

This is a short exercise that does not require any more action.

What makes it work better

If there is humour in the answers and/or responses.

What can go wrong

Some participants may feel threatened by the idea of an 'IQ' test and do not take it in the spirit in which it is intended.

INTELLIGENCE TEST (unknown source)

One minute only allowed

Write your name in the square provided.

If you were alone in a deserted house at night and there was a lamp, a fire and a candle and you only had one match, which would you light first?

If you drove a bus from London with 50 passengers and dropped off 8 and picked up 5 at Brighton, stopped at Southampton and picked up 5 and dropped off 13, and then drove to arrive in Edinburgh 11 hours later, what was the driver's name?

Some months have 31 days and some have 30 days, but how many have 28 days?

If a friend gave you five sweets and told you to take one every half hour, how long would they last?

Divide 50 by $\frac{1}{2}$ and add 10.

Which country has a Fourth of July – the UK or the USA?

If you take three pears from four pears, what do you have?

Write your name here.

Answers to INTELLIGENCE TEST

Write your name in the square provided.	Participant should have written this in the square at the bottom of the page.
If you were alone in a deserted house at night and there was a lamp, a fire and a candle and you only had one match, which would you light first?	The match
If you drove a bus from London with 50 passengers and dropped off 8 and picked up 5 at Brighton, stopped at Southampton and picked up 5 and dropped off 13, and then drove to arrive in Edinburgh 11 hours later, what was the driver's name?	Participant should have written their own name
Some months have 31 days and some have 30 days, but how many have 28 days?	All months
If a friend gave you five sweets and told you to take one every half hour, how long would they last?	Two hours
Divide 50 by ½ and add 10.	110
Which country has a Fourth of July – the UK or the USA?	Both
If you take three pears from four pears, what do you have?	Three pears
	Name written here

18

Accessing, assessing and using information management

Our environment is changing constantly, and what we need to know changes with it. Sometimes we assimilate a gradual shift without realising that we are altering the way in which we do things, and we acquire the information that is needed in a steady way. More often we need to make specific efforts to identify what it is that we do not know and to put in place the remedies.

In order to avoid having to make sudden unpleasant jumps from where we are to where we should be, we need to evaluate our level of knowledge and skills on a continuous basis.[1] Think about how you establish and maintain the following:

- in-house formal education and training
- individual learning projects
- workplace or organisational learning projects
- methods of assessing learning records and achievements
- support facilities for learning.

Accurate data

Evaluating how you are performing and the gaps in your provision, knowledge or skills depends on being able to extract the relevant information from your data. Reliable and accurate data depend on:

- entering data once
- entering data consistently and correctly
- being able to retrieve data for a variety of uses
- being able to compare the data with others.

To use data effectively, we need to connect information systems to one another and to make retrieval easy. For example, best practice integrates clinical information systems with readily available information on clinical guidelines and relevant research, as well as epidemiology, audit and evaluation databases. We also require patient and professional education and information and quality assessment tools that are accessible to both professional and patient. Electronic records make each part of the information open to different levels of access, supplement information that is not easily available by other means (e.g. waiting times), and can be consulted remotely across large distances.

Training issues

Acquiring information technology skills is often assumed to be an optional add-on for people who are interested in the subject. However, learning how to enhance your skills makes access to continuous learning much easier.[2] Training for all staff should:

- be based on the needs of the participants
- be available to all staff
- be based at work if possible and take place in working time
- encompass multidisciplinary working
- reflect the wide variety of systems in use.

Parallel training in the critical assessment of the quality of information sources helps people to select the data or information source that is most relevant to the task. When technology is introduced, think about how to:

- minimise the training needed to use it
- prevent security measures being circumvented
- record/retrieve information at the right time in a standard way (all staff should know how to use IT)
- incorporate audit and risk management
- base decisions on accurate information.

Anybody who designs a system for storing data, or who is required to put the data into such a system, has a responsibility to:

- know the purpose for which the data are being entered
- have a common understanding of how the data will be recorded
- understand the limitations of any data extracted, the criteria used and the factors that influence the result
- make requests to extract data that are precise and clearly defined, or the results will be inaccurate or, worse, misleading
- be explicit about data input for any new working practice or developments
- understand the processes involved in that workplace or organisation as well as to know how the information is stored. There is a misconception that information analysis can be undertaken by anyone, even without training or a good grasp of the complexities involved.

How you could demonstrate the benefits of information management in a learning culture

The first objective is to establish an area where change is recognised as necessary and accepted (*see* Chapter 12). Implementing a change based on research evidence can be a useful learning experience and can demonstrate to a team or organisation the importance of accessing, assessing and using information. Tips gained from others[3] include the following.

- Select a topic for which the evidence is conclusive and convincing.
- Enlist the support of key people who support the change, have local credibility and are willing to promote and argue for the change.
- Focus on an area that will make a visible change and be welcomed, ideally by patients, staff and managers.
- Tie in your change with local priorities and opportunities.
- Identify the best (but readily available) indicators of the impact or outcome in order to measure these before, during and after the lifespan of the work. You may need to be pragmatic about what can be measured.
- Exploit any natural links with other priorities and initiatives.
- Make the link with training, audit and reflective practice.
- Everyone who will be involved needs to be identified, involved and informed.
- Tackle something realistic and achievable.

Assessing and evaluating sources of information and research

Time and resources are necessary ingredients for reflecting on what you are doing now, obtaining the relevant information about what others are doing for comparison, and evaluating the usefulness of new information about what might be done in the future.

When trying to evaluate in this way, it is important to recognise the following points.

- Consider that any one piece of information, snapshot of performance or study focuses on only a small corner of the world. The information has to be taken in context and judged for its relevance to the wider world.
- As the critical evaluator, separate out the broad aim of the study and the precise objectives, and do not assess the study for what it did not set out to do.

- Appraise the way in which the study has been conducted or the information collected.
- Reflect on the broader purpose, relevance and implications of the study or information. In particular, think about how it applies to your own work or organisation.
- Identify the clear results and reflect on what the less clear results show. No study or collection of data is ever perfect, and it is important to recognise that this is an impossible dream. We must make the most of what we have, 'warts and all'.
- Acknowledge that statistical analysis can be useful, but logic and common sense are more important.

Sources of information

The lack of access to computers connected to each other or to the Internet can be a physical barrier (not enough computer terminals in the right place) or due to a lack of skill in accessing the information available. More and more guidelines, clinical standards, recommendations and other information are becoming available, and staff need to be able to use computer networks to access them. Hardware and software need to be readily available and easy to use, and the development of skills to use them should be encouraged.

In some areas[4] initiatives have included the following:

- searching for clinical and non-clinical information that is available to all and supported by library staff
- courses in effective literature searching that are run regularly. This might be extended to include basic statistical training, basic research methodology, and decision-tree analysis. Critical appraisal courses that are run on-site can focus on local problems identified by local teams, and can progress at the right pace for that team
- home pages on the intranet for the workplace or organisation can include information and access to distance-learning projects
- the establishment of a computer-assisted learning centre that is networked on an intranet so that services such as research information, textbook and training information are available to all staff from any terminal.

Sources of information are changing all the time. Using an Internet site with links to many others takes the tedium out of searching for relevant material. There are many of these, so find one that you like and use it to access other sources of information.

References

1 Wakley G, Chambers R and Field S (2000) *Continuing Professional Development in Primary Care: making it happen.* Radcliffe Medical Press, Oxford.

2 Kinn S and Jones R (1995) Continuing education in health informatics in the UK: the need for learning materials. *Medinfo.* **8**: 1260–4.

3 Evans D (2000) Top tips for implementing changes in practice based on research evidence. *Clin Govern Bull.* **1**: 6.

4 Donnald A (1998) *The Front Line Evidence Base Medicine Project: final report.* NHS Executive North Thames Regional Office, Research and Development, London.

Games, activities and learning techniques

Exercise 18.1 Keeping a reflective learning log

Why you should do this

Participants should have a permanent record of their learning to keep in their portfolios. It can then be extracted at a later date if evidence of learning activities is required for supervision, appraisal or accreditation.

When to use this

You might use this exercise over a series of workshops when the content is very unstructured and few handouts will be available. For example, it might be used in conjunction with the Oslo technique (*see* Exercise 16.2) or when the objectives of the workshop have been changed in response to feedback (*see* Exercises in Chapter 9).

It can also be used as a stand-alone exercise to support other learning that will be discussed or reviewed with a mentor, coach or tutor.

What to do

Give some guidance on what sort of record you are expecting. For example:

The purpose of the learning log is for participants to pick out the most personally significant experiences on a particular day and record what they learned from those experiences. This will involve reflecting on:
• what was most significant
• why this was personally significant
• what you learned
• any actions you propose to take as a result.

You need not restrict yourself to one event. You can also use the log to record other thoughts, ideas, insights and feelings. In addition, you might also record what worked for you and what did not, and the reasons for this. Other observations might include the relevance of the learning to your work or personal life.

How it works (insight)

This exercise helps participants to reflect on the significance to them of what and how they are learning. They become more aware of both of these aspects of their learning.

Whom to engage

Any group or individual. This approach has been used successfully for augmenting seminar learning of skills in counselling and psychoanalytical work, but it requires time for review.

How much time you should allow

If you are doing this exercise in a series of workshops, set aside time to complete the logbook at the end of each session. This emphasises the importance that you attach to the task. The participants will need about 30 minutes per half day of learning activities.

It is unrealistic to expect anyone to spend more time than this on a regular basis if used for unstructured learning.

What the facilitator should do

Make the task completely clear, and be ready to help novices to start recording their reflections about their learning. Allocate sufficient time for the completion of the logs as well as time for review and reflection. Encourage those individuals who are reluctant to commit their thoughts to paper.

What to do next

Suggest that the participants might find this a useful technique for reflecting on other learning activities. Encourage them to look at their learning styles and to consider whether other ways of working might suit them better.

What makes it work better

- Practise reflecting about learning and work.
- Self-motivated learners who are keen to progress.

What can go wrong

- People who have been sent on courses or who are reluctant learners and so do not want to spend time reflecting on their learning.
- A culture of 'going off to the pub for socialising' after learning.
- People who squeeze learning in between other activities which they perceive to be more important, and who rush off home or back to work without allowing time for reflection.

Exercise 18.2 Thinking hats

Why you should do this

It helps participants to identify their own and other people's thinking and learning styles (*see* Chapter 1).

When to use this

In any situation where participants need to develop problem solving and evaluative skills.

What to do

Explain each of the hats:

- *the research and observation hat*: observe and question people, and then choose a course of action based on your own observations
- *the many-crowned hat*: work out several different ways of approaching the task, and then modify and improve the one that seems most promising
- *the pointed hat*: fix your direction firmly and concentrate on solving the problem by a thorough application of this approach
- *the experiential hat*: work out an approach based on things that worked in the past, avoiding those that did not work in the past
- *the flexible step-at-a-time hat*: work out the approach one step at a time, reconsidering each step as you come to it, and altering direction if necessary in a flexible way
- *the playful hat*: play with the ideas freely, brainstorm, and apply whatever turns up.

Divide the participants into small groups of not less than three in each group. Each group takes a hat and a written prepared task. If there are not enough people, use only some of the hats, and have a second round using the other hats, or ask the participants to try out two of the hats. Return to the plenary group for a brief presentation from each small group, and then discuss how the different hats were used.

How it works (insight)

It demonstrates that when tasks are approached in different ways, there is an increased likelihood of innovative or interesting solutions. It encourages the participants to investigate other ways of looking at tasks, and to appreciate other people's approaches. Problem solving becomes a more interesting challenge.

Whom to engage

Groups in which members will have to make action plans or manage situations.

How much time you should allow

Allow about 10 minutes for the explanations, about 30 minutes for the small groups, 5 minutes each for feedback and 25 minutes for the general discussion.

What the facilitator should do

Find some amusing hats. For example:

- a hat with glasses on for the research and observation one
- a jester's hat for the many-crowned one
- a witch's hat for the pointed one
- a hard hat for the experiential one
- a hat that can be changed – with side flaps or a roll-down flap – for the flexible step-at-a-time one
- a fantasy hat for the playful one.

Write the explanations on a card to go with each hat. Provide tasks that are relevant to the group members (e.g. how adult learners can get more out of education, or how we can find time to learn). Keep to time and move people on if they seem to be getting stuck.

What to do next

Draw conclusions about how people used the hats. Ask them for illustrations of how they might apply what they have learned to other situations, or to the activities that follow.

What makes it work better

Groups who are prepared to be flexible and to adopt the method suggested.

What can go wrong

Groups may adhere rigidly to methods that they have always used, and find it difficult to appreciate other ways of working.

Exercise 18.3 Bits of books

Why you should do this

It enables small groups to work quickly together gathering information.

When to use this

To introduce people to looking critically at written sources of information.

What to do

Divide the group into smaller syndicate groups of at least four people. Give enough pages of the publication to allow each participant 1–3 pages depending on the content and density of the print. Tell them that they have to speed read the pages in a fixed time, summarise the contents mentally or jot them down, and then explain to each other the content of their pages. Ask each syndicate group to prepare a list on an acetate sheet for an overhead projector or to write on a piece of paper what is important from the pages that they have. Then each group presents their list. The whole group then discusses whether the sense of the publication has been obtained, if not why not, and how this type of task could be delegated to a group.

How it works (insight)

This exercise encourages people who would not otherwise read critically to recognise that this is a skill that can be readily learned. It illustrates how quickly people can get a flavour of what something is about, and how easy it is to misunderstand information if one does not have a complete picture.

Whom to engage

Participants who think that they have no time to read, or that books and other publications are something that other people read.

How much time you should allow

This depends somewhat on the level of literacy in the group. Professionals who are used to speed reading can read two or three pages very quickly and summarise them in about 5 minutes. Others who are less used to reading may take 10 minutes. Allow about 10 minutes for presentations in the syndicate groups and drawing up the list, and about 30 minutes for the discussion in the large group before drawing conclusions.

What the facilitator should do

Photocopy or tear up a booklet containing a report about an innovation or introduction of a new service, or a short government publication. If you are uncertain about the variations in literacy or comprehension levels of some of your participants in a multidisciplinary workshop, use something more general such as a tourist information brochure. Make sure that the publication is long enough for each person to have a complete section. You will need to duplicate pages that have sentences which go over the page and cross out what has gone before or afterwards.

Keep people to time, and bring the general discussion to a close when the points of agreement and disagreement have been made – do not allow them to go on until the substance of the publication is clearly understood by everyone!

What to do next

Use the misconceptions and the summary lists to illustrate the points and suggest ways in which the participants might apply the learning to other situations.

What makes it work better

People who are used to summarising documents will do the task quickly, but will also include more misconceptions.

What can go wrong

- The presentation in the plenary group can become quite heated as misconceptions appear.
- People may argue about the meaning of the document and get bogged down by explaining the errors.

Exercise 18.4 Resources

Why you should do this

To widen people's knowledge of where information can be obtained.

When to use this

For introducing ideas about adult learning or about self-motivation for learning, or as a break from more intense activities.

What to do

Spread out around the room a selection of research papers, printouts from websites, information booklets, books, sources of information on the Internet, etc. Make sure that everyone has a pad of paper and pen. Allow the participants time to wander around the room making notes about anything that interests them.

You can increase their involvement by asking each participant to bring along an interesting paper, publication, book or page from a website.

After the time is up, invite comments on the usefulness of the exercise.

How it works (insight)

This exercise introduces the participants to a range of materials and resources of which they may have been unaware. It helps people to recognise the types of information sources that they would find helpful.

Whom to engage

Groups who are new to learning or who have little experience of self-motivated learning.

How much time you should allow

Allow at least 30 to 45 minutes. If the participants are looking bored and start talking among themselves, you may need to bring them back more quickly and discuss why they found the exercise unhelpful.

What the facilitator should do

Identify as many of the likely interests of the participants as possible. Print out relevant pages from websites and ensure that the source is marked. Similarly, it should be clear where any research paper was published. Ensure that all of the rcsources brought are clearly marked with the owners' names, and offer to photocopy any that people want to take away with them (or they will disappear).

What to do next

If your focus is on resources for learning, a talk with a handout from an expert might be useful.

What makes it work better

Materials applicable to the interests of the participants that they have not already seen.

What can go wrong

The participants may not be interested in the resources, or may not think that they will want to seek any out such sources of information for themselves.

19

Under-performance

Under-performance is an important issue for organisations because it:

- detracts from the organisation achieving its goals
- can put both personnel and clients at risk
- can contribute towards an unhealthy culture within the organisation
- can be a source of stress for staff who work with an under-performing individual.

It is also an important issue for the individual, as it can lead to stress, failure to realise their full potential and job dissatisfaction.

What is under-performance?

Under-performance can cover a range of issues, such as knowledge, skills, behaviour and attitudes. It is about achieving less than expectations, or performing below the required levels. Under-performance can be defined in terms of accepted local, professional or national standards (i.e. when performance fails to meet explicit required standards). It can also be defined in terms of relative performance, where the performance of the individual concerned is that of an outlier compared with the performance of his or her peers. Sometimes under-performance is defined in terms of consistently placing patients or customers at risk.

A single incident will not normally constitute under-performance, but repeated less important infringements may do so.

Causes of under-performance

Individuals who under-perform may:

- be generally passive
- be fearful of challenge and avoid it whenever possible
- avoid seeking insight into themselves and their beliefs
- find feedback and criticism threatening
- have low reserves of energy

- have poor motivation
- resent others' success
- fail to realise their potential.

Sometimes the problem arises from a malfunctioning organisation such as:

- poor management of quality processes
- inadequate infrastructure and insufficient resources to undertake tasks
- poor communication within the work setting
- an unhealthy culture within the organisation
- a culture of fear and lack of openness
- inappropriate styles of management and organisational structure.

Diagnosing under-performance

One of the commonest ways of diagnosing under-performance is when a manager perceives that the individual is not performing at their expected levels or their attitude is inappropriate. This may be based either on qualitative measures such as failure to achieve certain targets, or on a quantitative assessment of aspects of their performance. This might be relative to others, such as an individual or organisation consistently performing below the level of peers.

Sometimes it is the level or nature of complaints that indicates under-performance of an individual or organisation, or an individual may recognise that they or their organisation are under-performing and seek assistance.

Investigations of cases of possible under-performance should be:

- specific to the individual concerned
- related to the area of concern
- measurable (with agreed methods of measurement)
- based on agreed indicators
- clear, simple and understood
- within well-defined time scales.

Tackling under-performance in individuals

Once under-performance has been recognised, the solutions will depend on the diagnosis. The range of interventions for an individual could include the following:

- providing support through mentorship
- reassessment of training and development needs and programmes to meet these needs

- external independent assessment and advice on action
- agreeing on short-term action plans with performance targets (this may be on a daily or weekly basis in some instances)
- a programme to build self-esteem and assertiveness
- training programmes to change attitudes
- changing the environment to suit the needs of the individual
- formal disciplinary measures used as a last resort or reserved for serious cases.

Tackling under-performance in organisations

Identifying the type of problem helps to suggest remedies. Common problems that develop in organisations include the following.

- *Managers who do not manage but continue to operate as 'workers'.* A manager is not just responsible for him- or herself, but for the results obtained by a group of people. People who are talented at their own work do not always see the necessity for learning 'people skills' to motivate and manage others, and may need training to improve their skills.
- *Failure to delegate.* A project that may seem overwhelming if you do it by yourself becomes achievable if the tasks are divided between people in a team who will be responsible for each part. Skills in learning how to delegate and trusting people to attend to the detail while you keep the overall direction on course have to be learned.
- *No clear targets set.* If managers do not make the ultimate and intermediate goals obvious, others have no idea where they are going. Being in a rudderless ship – appearing to drift along – reduces motivation and drive.
- *Poor communication.* The larger the organisation, the greater the need for formal lines of communication to make sure that everyone is informed and rumours are not allowed to develop.
- *Rigid attitudes.* People become used to doing things in a certain way. When the organisation's environment changes, managers need to be constantly trying new methods of coping with the new circumstances. Leaders who resist change prevent workplace teams from learning new ways of functioning.
- *Managers who are not available to their colleagues and subordinates.* Some people need little support or supervision. Others, particularly when new in an organisation, need a lot. If you manage a team, but never find time to enquire about its members' needs, or to focus on what they have to say, they will become embittered and resentful, and will cease to work efficiently.

- *Failing to acknowledge achievements.* If all that the leadership does is pile on more work, no one will do a good job. The quality of the work and the time and effort put in have to be seen to have a value for the work to continue to be worthwhile.
- *Going for the quick fix rather than understanding and finding solutions that will work in the longer term.* The immediate and obvious solution is usually wrong because the implications of that change have not been thought through. Further changes are then necessary and people start to doubt that anything will improve.
- *Never having any fun.* An organisation that always takes itself seriously and is targeted on achievement alone will lose the goodwill of its constituent parts.

Further reading

Rotherham G, Martin D, Joesbury H and Mathers N (1997) *Measures to Assist GPs Whose Performance Gives Cause for Concern.* School of Health and Related Research, University of Sheffield, Sheffield.

Games, activities and learning techniques

Exercise 19.1 Listening but not hearing

Why you should do this

To explore the feelings generated by not listening to someone and to demonstrate the powerful technique of 'mirroring', where an individual actively mirrors the body language, eye contact, tone of voice, types of words used and even breathing, etc., of the person with whom he or she is communicating.

When to use this

In a workshop.

What to do

1 Divide the workshop members into pairs labelled A and B, respectively.
2 Ask the As to describe to their partners, in no more than 5 minutes, their last major holidays.
3 The Bs should sit opposite their partners who are describing their holidays, but actively try not to hear what they are saying. They can do anything except leave the chair.

4   After 5 minutes the As are asked to repeat their holiday stories to their partners.
5   This time the Bs mirror their partners and actively listen to what they are saying. They should respond in the same tone of voice, copy their posture, maintain eye contact and body language, etc.
6   A and B then switch roles and B tells A about their holiday and they repeat the two stages described above.
7   The participants then reconvene as a plenary group and discuss what feelings were generated by the speaker in the first half of the exercise compared with the second half, when their partners were mirroring them.

How it works (insight)

One of the commonest complaints made by individuals who are diagnosed as under-performing is that their seniors do not listen to their concerns. This exercise demonstrates the effects of not listening and provides a practical method for improving listening skills.

Whom to engage

Those who wish to improve their communication and listening skills.

How much time you should allow

This exercise could take 40 to 60 minutes depending on the amount of discussion that ensues.

What the facilitator should do

The facilitator should explain the purpose of the exercise and the basics of the mirroring technique. Space the pairs out round the room. Help participants to keep to time for the listening and mirroring exercises.

What to do next

Practise mirroring and active listening in everyday working life, and report back on progress at a future date.

What makes it work better

The person who is designated as the 'listener' adopts all kinds of behaviour to make it obvious that they are not 'hearing' their partner who is telling them about his or her holiday in the first round. For example, they could fidget in their chair, pick up a book and thumb through it, hum, or look away at another part of the room.

What can go wrong

The person who is designated as the 'listener' may not distinguish sufficiently between 'not hearing' and 'mirroring' their partner.

Exercise 19.2 Television slot

Why you should do this

To allow expression of a person's strengths.

When to use this

Towards the end of a workshop or within a team.

What to do

1 Divide the workshop into teams of three or four people.
2 Instruct each team to prepare a series of 2-minute television presentations (adverts or documentary style) for each member of the team.
3 The presentation needs to sell to the audience as many positive features as possible about that person – their experience, skills, personality, strengths, other attributes, achievements, etc., and to make an impact.
4 Each team of four people prepares a set of four 2-minute presentations.
5 Team members other than the individual it is about should perform the television presentation in front of the plenary group.

How it works (insight)

Under-performance can be exacerbated by continual criticism and focusing on weaknesses. In this exercise, each individual can demonstrate their strengths and achievements without involving themselves personally in the final presentation.

Whom to engage

Anyone and everyone.

How much time you should allow

It will take 10 to 15 minutes to prepare each advert, so allow 60 to 80 minutes to prepare and perform four television presentations. If there are three groups of four people, then an additional 40 minutes will be required for presentations.

What the facilitator should do

Explain the objectives of the exercise and establish teams of three or four people. Teams could be allocated randomly, or if there is a wide range of experience or seniority, allocate people to mix the groups. Provide a range of materials, such as flip charts, pens, overhead projector and transparencies. Tell each group when 15 minutes are up and they need to switch to preparing another presentation, and remind participants of the time if their presentations take too long.

What to do next

This is generally a 'feel-good' exercise, and the next session could look at weaknesses or areas for further development, etc.

What makes it work better

Some humour in the content of the presentations, so that the participants have fun working together on the task.

What can go wrong

Some of the participants who are presenting may not do justice to the subject of the presentation.

Exercise 19.3 A picture of under-performance

Why you should do this

To explore the nature of under-performance by focusing on a wide variety of causes. To think creatively about the problems and look at what under-performance means for management and for the organisation as a whole.

When to use this

For participants who are particularly interested in under-performance, or those with a general interest in management-related issues such as leadership, teamworking, etc.

What to do

Teams should create a relevant scenario of under-performance – the person who is under-performing, what his or her managers are like and what kind of organisation this person works in. The individuals should consider the causes of the under-performance as well as its impact.

1 Divide the larger group into teams of around five people.
2 Ask the teams to come up with a pictorial representation of the scenario as follows:
   •   what an under-performing individual is like (i.e. personal characteristics)
   •   what the management of this under-performing person is like
   •   what the organisation in whom this person works is like.
3 Advise the teams to start by considering each of these perspectives in turn, exploring the causes of under-performance and making a list of all of the issues that are raised. Drawing pictures from these ideas can be left towards the end of the exercise.
4 The pictures are then shared with the larger group, accompanied by brief commentaries.

How it works (insight)

This exercise allows participants to explore different stereotypes of the under-performing individual, and the management and organisation in which that individual works. It allows people to think creatively about the causes of under-performance and how it affects both the individual him- or herself and the organisation as a whole.

Whom to engage

All those involved in managing people, and particularly those who have an interest in managing difficult individuals.

How much time you should allow

Allow 45 minutes for developing the pictorial representation and then a maximum of 5 minutes for the presentation from each group.

What the facilitator should do

Ensure that flip charts and coloured pens are readily available for the team, and that there is an easy method of establishing small groups of five people. The facilitator should also try to ensure wherever possible that people from the same organisation/department are not present in the same group. Participants should be encouraged to think creatively about the causes of under-performance as well as its consequences.

Have one or two sample scenarios available in case participants have difficulty in creating their own.

What to do next

Various approaches to preventing and reversing under-performance could be explored in follow-up sessions.

What makes it work better

Basing the scenarios on actual cases may make the exercise more meaningful and help to solve outstanding problems.

What can go wrong

If a large number of participants come from the same department or organisation, there may be a danger that individuals are identifiable through the ensuing discussions.

20

Appraisal

Good employment practice includes regular job appraisal, at least annually. This gives you an opportunity to review how well you are doing in your own view and in that of the person who is appraising you. The two of you can agree on your learning needs and how they will be met in the context of your current job or agreed changes to your roles and responsibilities.

Most employees will have an arrangement for their work to be supervised by their manager. The supervision should be appropriate to their job situation and learning needs. If your field of work is specialised, a work colleague who is aware of the requirements of your post could provide supervision (e.g. supervision of clinical nursing duties could be arranged with a clinical tutor or supervisor).

Competencies or deficiencies in the quality of performance can be listed under the following three main areas:

• professional competence
• relationships with other people
• ethical standards.

Be pro-active and look at these areas critically both for yourself and for others working with you. It is best practice to use risk management to try to prevent failures before they occur.

Use the grid in Exercise 20.3 (*see* page 210) as an example of information that you might obtain either as an individual or as a group before an appraisal interview.

Professional competence

Whatever work you do, you should meet certain minimum individual professional standards. Unacceptable standards include being:

• unaware of the limits of your competence, or unwilling to ask for help when those limits are reached
• a poor listener, who misses important parts of communications made to you

- unable to discuss sensitive and personal underlying matters that affect others
- unable or unwilling to explain what you are going to do or why
- poorly organised to prevent future problems, give appropriate health or safety advice, or supervise long-term problems
- someone who undertakes or arranges irrelevant procedures or investigations
- someone who gives or arranges remedies or treatments that are not consistent with best practice or evidence.

A person who does not meet minimum acceptable standards also fails to:

- use previous records as a source of information about past events
- arrange examination when needed in an appropriate or adequate way
- have or use suitable equipment that is in working order
- follow rational and logical thought processes from the information available
- keep up to date with current legal or organisational developments
- maintain proper records and systems of review.

If you or someone you work with have any of these difficulties, look at the reasons in the same way as you would in a significant incident analysis. Decide with others whether it is an important enough problem or occurs sufficiently often to require remedial action.

Other deficiencies that may affect the performance of the whole team or workplace include the following.

1   People have difficulty accessing services because of:
    - restricted opening hours, or hours that are unpredictable
    - too few, unanswered or frequently engaged phone lines
    - unavailability of staff
    - poor, difficult or unsafe access to premises or parts of premises
    - lack of information about the services available.
2   People receive a poor quality of service because of:
    - inadequately trained staff or staff with poor levels of competence
    - lack of confidentiality
    - staff not being contactable or effective in an emergency
    - services being unavailable due to poor management of resources or services
    - insufficient numbers of available staff for the workload
    - the qualifications of deputising staff being unknown or inadequate for the posts that they are filling
    - the arrangements for transfer of information from one team member to another being inadequate
    - team members not acting on information received.

Many of these items will need action as a team, but for some of them it may be your responsibility to ensure that adequate standards are met.

Relationships with others

It is important that everyone feels that they can bring problems to the attention of others without fear of blame or giving or taking offence.

Other people should be treated with respect. Good communications are essential, and procedures for reliable transmission of messages should be in place.

Unacceptable standards for relationships with others include the following:

- prejudices against ethnic groups, the homeless, and those with severe mental illness or other conditions
- pressuring others to act in line with your own beliefs
- failing to provide safeguards for the staff when they have to see people who pose a threat to them
- having no contact with or refusing to talk to other members of the team
- failing to listen to people's concerns
- being unaware of the skills of others
- delegating tasks to inappropriately or inadequately trained staff
- failing to encourage staff to develop new skills and responsibilities
- failing to refer appropriately problems beyond your level of competence
- failing to provide sufficient information to others
- paying insufficient attention to confidentiality and consent.

Some of these items require action by an individual, while others require the whole team to make changes. Team meetings are often a good way of raising concerns at an early stage.

The team members can give 360° feedback to each other as part of annual appraisals. This means that colleagues who are junior to, peers of and senior to every person in the team will give him or her constructive feedback about his or her perceived performance. Such feedback may cover attitudes, timekeeping and general remarks, as well as referring to their knowledge and skills. This honest feedback should *enhance* and not *disrupt* the teambuilding. Usually such feedback is anonymised, but in small teams it is difficult to make remarks about people that cannot be attributed to individual informants.

Ethical standards

Some of the standards for professional competence and relationships with colleagues will also have ethical implications. Poor ethical standards may also be manifested by:

- giving references that are biased or untrue, or omitting important information

- signing or issuing certificates or documents that contain inaccurate information, or not considering their implications
- not taking responsibility for your actions or performance
- ignoring other people's unacceptable performance or behaviour
- seeking personal gain over and above the normal remuneration for your work
- misusing funds or abusing trust by inappropriate financial or personal dealings
- making poor use of the resources available
- failing to protect people from harm in research studies, or providing false data
- not taking proper responsibility for the quality of teaching when instructing others.

You may encounter other items not included in the above list, in which case you should add them to your criteria.

Useful reading

British Association of Medical Managers (1999) *Appraisal in Action: appraisal for hospital doctors.* British Association of Medical Managers, Stockport.

Edis M (1995) *Performance Management and Appraisal in Health Services.* Kogan Page, London.

Gatrell J and White T (2001) *Medical Appraisal, Selection and Revalidation.* The Royal Society of Medicine Press Ltd, London.

Haman H, Irvine S and Jelley D (2001) *The Peer Appraisal Handbook for General Practitioners.* Radcliffe Medical Press, Oxford.

Games, activities and learning techniques
Exercise 20.1 Team assessments

Why you should do this

This is a non-threatening way to start thinking about appraisal skills.

When to use this

After any activity that has involved a group of people, but particularly after learning tasks involving teambuilding or group co-operation.

What to do

Use prepared sheets for recording. Arrange participants in small groups. Invite them to reflect individually on the activity that has just been completed. Remind them about the rules for feedback (e.g. always make positive statements first) (*see* Chapter 1). Then they can share the reflections within the group, after which they meet back in the plenary group and the facilitator records the general conclusions of each syndicate group.

How it works (insight)

Participants gain confidence in their own ability to assess people's contributions within a team. As it is an artificially constituted team, criticisms are not as personal as they would be in a group where people have well-established roles. This gives people more freedom to be frank.

Whom to engage

Any group consisting of people from diverse backgrounds.

How much time you should allow

Allow 10 minutes for individual reflection, 10 to 15 minutes for the small group discussion (depending on how many people there are in the group), and 20 to 30 minutes for the plenary session at the end.

What the facilitator should do

Prepare a recording sheet suitable for assessing the team behaviour in the previous activity. Possible questions might include the following.

- What contribution did you make?
- What contributions did others make?
- What else could you or others have done to make it work better?
- What barriers to teamworking emerged?
- How did you feel about the activity?
- What do you think others were feeling and why do you think this?
- How can you apply what you have learned from this activity?

Make sure that you keep the conclusions general and applicable to the situations under consideration. Rephrase any personal comments. For example, change (with a smile) 'Y was very bossy' to 'I understand that X thought that Y adopted an autocratic leadership role – do others in that group think this was useful?'

What to do next

If there were many difficulties, the discussion could be extended to a more general review of how to make assessments, the rules of feedback, communication difficulties, etc. (*see* Chapters 3 to7).

What makes it work better

A group of people who are sensitive enough to others' feelings to phrase things carefully, but comfortable enough in the group to be frank.

What can go wrong

Participants may make personal and negative remarks about each other.

Exercise 20.2 Setting criteria for appraisal

Why you should do this

It helps participants to understand better what they are looking for if they are appraising someone else, or what they should prepare if they themselves are being appraised.

When to use this

For people who are either learning how to appraise others, or who have anxieties about appraisal procedures that are being introduced. Use it after a preliminary discussion or talk on giving feedback (*see* Chapter 1).

What to do

Divide the group into three syndicate groups, and give each of them one of the following sections to work on:

- professional competence
- relationships with other people
- ethical standards.

1 Give each syndicate group the heading and written instructions. Run through the written instructions and ask whether the participants have any questions.
2 Ask each participant to write down individually three to five criteria for their section.

3 The syndicate group then discusses the criteria, clarifies them and ranks them in order of importance.

4 Meet back as a large group. Record the criteria under the headings in the order in which the group has ranked them. In order to keep everyone's attention, have three flip-chart sheets visible and take one criterion from each group in turn.

5 Then ask if anyone can add any other criteria. Suggest any yourself if you think that there are criteria missing, explaining why you feel that they should be added, and allowing group discussion before adding them to the list.

6 With the large group, put the criteria into clusters and weed out any duplication.

7 Give each criterion a letter of the alphabet. Ask each participant, working individually, to rank them with a scoring system. Tell them that they have 30 points to give in total, and that they should allocate points (from one upwards) to each criterion according to how important they feel that it is. They can allocate zero if they personally feel that this criterion should not be included in the list.

8 Go through the criteria one by one collecting the scores. Add them up (you may need a calculator!).

9 Discuss the ratings and the reasons for any variations between scorers.

How it works (insight)

This allows people to see how the criteria for appraisal might be formulated. It gives them confidence to challenge any criteria which they feel are unsuitable or unfair. It also provides them with a sense of ownership and understanding of the criteria.

Whom to engage

People who are concerned with or about appraisal procedures.

How much time you should allow

This is a long exercise, and you will need to allow about 2 to 2½ hours in total. The approximate times for each of the nine sections are as follows:

1 2–5 minutes
2 8–10 minutes
3 20–30 minutes
4 15 minutes
5 15 minutes
6 5–10 minutes

7   20–25 minutes (it is a hard task!)
8   5–10 minutes
9   20–30 minutes.

What the facilitator should do

Prepare your own list of required criteria from various sources. Prepare three sheets with the headings and, on a separate sheet, a copy of the instructions for each participant. Keep to time, and encourage everyone to participate and contribute. Make suggestions only when it is clear that the group has missed out something significant. Guard against the session becoming one in which you as the expert tell the group what criteria to include. Make sure that there is enough room for participants to work individually without collusion.

What to do next

You might compare the list of criteria and the weightings given with one or two examples from the literature, and discuss the reasons for the variations. This exercise can usefully lead on to work on interviewing skills.

What makes it work better

Participants with some (but not too much) experience in appraisal or supervision.

What can go wrong

If there are a few people in the group who have a lot of experience and are not flexible in their approach, they may become entrenched in their opinions and unable to see how others might disagree with them, causing irritation to other group members or, worse, passive acceptance of the dominant opinions.

Exercise 20.3   Building up appraisal skills

Why you should do this

It increases people's ability to understand how to assess written material.

When to use this

With people who are starting to train in appraisal techniques, or who are anxious about the introduction of appraisal.

What to do

1 Divide the group into smaller syndicate groups of four to five people. Give the same prepared fictional or anonymised preparation sheet for an appraisal interview to each group. Warn them that one person will need to present back to the plenary group on the marking grid, and another on the list of questions for the subject.
2 Ask the groups to draw up a marking grid with criteria on a flip-chart sheet (*see* page 210 for an example). Suggest that they might use a Likert scale ranging from 'well shown' to 'poorly shown', or 'yes/no' marking, whichever is more appropriate.
3 The groups mark the sample preparation sheet.
4 They then prepare a list of questions that they would like to ask the subject of the preparation sheet.
5 In the plenary group, ask one member from each syndicate group to present their marking.
6 Compare and discuss the marking schemes.
7 In the large group, ask one member from each syndicate group to present their questions.
8 Compare and discuss the questions.
9 Allow a little time for summing up and general discussion of people's feelings about the exercise.

How it works (insight)

It allows participants to practise appraisal skills, and makes people feel more confident in their ability both to be appraised fairly and to appraise others.

Whom to engage

Groups that have done some preparatory work on giving feedback, or before or after a session on interviewing skills.

How much time you should allow

Allow about 45 to 50 minutes for the presentation of the task, dividing into groups, reviewing the prepared sheet, drawing up the grid and preparing a list of questions. Give each group only 5 minutes to present the grid and marks, and then allow discussion for about 20 minutes. Again allow each group 5 minutes to present the list of questions and then discuss these for 20 minutes. Allow about 10 minutes at the end for general discussion. This is a long exercise – with four syndicate groups it takes about 2½ hours.

Example of a grid drawn up by a group for assessment of information obtained before an appraisal interview

Activity	Adequate standards shown	Some queries	Needs exploring	No information given
Clinical and/or working practice (e.g. video, log diary, significant event audit, patient feedback, colleague feedback, administrative audit, etc.)				
Maintaining good practice and learning (e.g. learning record, review of external learning courses, internal learning activity, etc.)				
Relationships with patients, staff and colleagues (e.g. formal and informal feedback, significant event audit, referral audit, etc.)				
Teaching/training others (e.g. formal and informal feedback, impact on patients and services, etc.)				
Probity and performance (e.g. giving references, implementing new research or guidelines, review of personal fitness for work, etc.)				

What the facilitator should do

Prepare or anonymise a preparation sheet for an appraisal interview. You may need to explain a Likert scale if people are not familiar with the concept. Prepare your own list of criteria and suggested questions so that you can prompt the participants if necessary. Keep to time and keep it light-hearted – it is hard work!

What to do next

You could compare the results from the group with other examples from publications. You may want to move on to consider feedback or interviewing skills in more detail. You might hear from one or two people who are experienced in appraisal or supervision how they do it.

What makes it work better

A group that is willing to work hard, and for whom the task is important or urgent.

What can go wrong

- Participants may feel that they have no control over the process, so they question why they should work at it.
- People who have rigid ideas about how appraisal should be done, and who try to impose these ideas on others.

21

Interviews and interviewing

This chapter applies equally well to teachers themselves and to learners. These days of frequent change and upheaval in the health service provide many opportunities for health professionals and managers to expand or change the direction of their careers.

Some people are always on the look-out for a better job which more closely suits their needs. Being pro-active means being aware of where you want to be in three to five years' time, what your strengths and weaknesses are, and what kind of job situation will best match your 'assets' and aspirations.

The games, activities and learning techniques which complete the chapter should enable teachers and learners of any level of seniority to benefit through feedback from other participants whilst they are practising via role play in a non-threatening learning environment.

Curriculum vitae (CV)

Your CV must:

- be well organised so that your strengths are well presented
- be clear and understandable with no spelling mistakes
- be of appropriate length for the position – usually no longer than two to three sides of A4 paper, although it may be appropriate to have a lengthier CV for a senior post
- not have gaps with regard to previous posts with dates. However, do not give too much detail about earlier years which would swamp more interesting current information
- describe the main job functions you have undertaken, your main achievements, and the training and skills that you have acquired.

Include a covering letter with your application that summarises how your experience, qualifications and interests match the most important job requirements of the post for which you are applying.

The interview

Spend plenty of time preparing for the interview. Make sure that you have all the details you need about the organisation to which you are applying and the job you will be required to do. Be able to describe your strengths and give illustrative examples. If you are asked about your weaknesses, think of one that might also be construed as a strength (e.g. humility), or which can be easily rectified by experience of working in the new post.

Ask a sympathetic partner or friend whom you trust to give you constructive feedback, and to let you practise with a mock interview.

Make a great first impression when you enter the room for the interview. The choice of applicant may be strongly swayed by their appearance, body language and voice in the first 60 seconds or so. The panel will be looking for someone who:

- is confident but not arrogant
- is pleasant and able to fit in within the workplace setting
- is serious about the job
- is energetic
- is thoughtful
- is punctual
- is motivated
- has good communications skills
- is reliable
- is honest
- has integrity
- is a teamworker.

Some questions are predictable, such as the following.

- Why do you want to work here?
- What experience do you have that is relevant to this job?
- What aspects of your current job fit you for this post?
- What are your strengths (give examples) and weaknesses?
- What skills do you bring to the team?
- Give an example from your previous career which shows that you have initiative.
- How have you contributed towards teamwork?

You will usually be given an opportunity to ask questions at the end of the interview, so use this to make a good impression. Ask questions that show your interests (opportunities for further developments, etc.).

After the interview

If you are offered the job, you may be able to negotiate some of the terms and conditions, such as the salary.

If you are unsuccessful, ask for feedback to find out why.

- Was it your CV?
- Was it how the interview went?
- Was it your lack of experience, skills or attitude?
- Will there be other opportunities to apply for similar or related positions?

Games, activities and learning techniques

Exercise 21.1 Predicting the future

Why you should do this

To enable participants to take a holistic approach when reviewing their past career and planning where they would like their future career to go. It could be used for personal development, and would be particularly useful for honing interview skills.

When to use this

In situations where personal and professional development is regarded as important, such as a tutorial or mentoring programme, or as a one-off workshop or one in a series of seminars.

What to do

1 Each participant takes a sheet of flip-chart paper and draws a line across the middle of the paper.
2 They then draw a circle in the middle of the line to represent the current time. The line starts at the time of their birth and finishes at the time of their death. Participants start from their birth and highlight key events that have occurred which have shaped their life. Such key events could be social, external, life events, etc. They then predict key events that will occur in the future and identify them on the time line.
3 Put up each participant's piece of flip-chart paper on the walls of the room with Blu-Tack, and encourage the group to look at other people's time lines and the different approaches that they have used to predict events.

How it works (insight)

This exercise gives those participating an opportunity to take stock of their lives and to gain insight into life and career planning.

Whom to engage

Individuals in training grades or established professionals who want to extend or change their careers.

How much time you should allow

A total of 30 minutes should be adequate.

What the facilitator should do

Explain the process. Have plenty of flip-chart paper and pens available. Provide Blu-Tack or other material to attach the papers to the walls. Encourage a supportive atmosphere if the exercise is undertaken as a group activity, so that no one mocks or judges others.

What to do next

Use the review together with other material for making personal development plans. Make action plans to work towards the desired future achievements.

What makes it work better

- People can share their work in pairs or small groups of four or five people instead of displaying the completed sheets of paper on the walls.
- Showing an example of the facilitator's own time line to illustrate what is required.

What can go wrong

- Participants who may have experienced distressing events in the past may become upset.
- Unthinking participants might mock or judge others' work.
- Someone who already feels alien to the group may feel even more separated from the others if their time lines are very different.

Exercise 21.2 Mock interviewing for a mystery job

Why you should do this

To defuse trainees' or students' fears about being interviewed, and to illustrate the similar characteristics that an interview panel seeks for all kinds of jobs (e.g. commitment, motivation, energy, etc.).

When to use this

As a fun exercise in a workshop with a group.

What to do

1 Volunteers form an interview panel of three or four people and an interview candidate.
2 The interview candidate leaves the room for a few minutes whilst the panel decides on the type of job and who will ask what questions.
3 The candidate should invent his or her past experience, skills, etc.
4 The panel should ask questions in such a way that they do not reveal the nature of the job too early in the exercise.
5 The 'candidate' returns to be interviewed, but he or she does not know what the job is! At the end of the interview, the candidate guesses what job he or she has just been interviewed for.
6 The interview should last for about 15 to 20 minutes. Following the interview, the panel members decide whether the candidate has been successful or not and give the reasons for their decision.
7 The exercise can be repeated with other volunteers.
8 A general discussion follows a number of these interview exercises, and considers what types of common characteristics are required by organisations for many jobs, and interview techniques (what works and what does not).

How it works (insight)

Not knowing the nature of the job makes the exercise fun to do, particularly if unusual jobs are chosen.

Whom to engage

This exercise is relevant to people who are seeking experience in conducting interviews as well as those who are expecting to attend interviews. It can also be used as part of a leadership programme to discuss the characteristics required in today's working environment.

How much time you should allow

Each interview will take around 15 to 20 minutes, so if there are three interviews followed by a 30-minute discussion, the total time will be around 90 minutes.

What the facilitator should do

The facilitator should give clear instructions to the interview panel and the candidate. They should place three or four chairs and a desk in front of the audience so that they can watch the interview, and they should provide the interview panel with paper and pens.

What to do next

Use the exercise to trigger discussion about today's job environment and the requirements of organisations.

What makes it work better

- For a more productive exercise, the panel could choose realistic jobs for which members of the audience would be likely to apply.
- While the candidate is out of the room and the panel are selecting an occupation, the audience could be informed from the beginning about the nature of the 'mystery job'.

What can go wrong

- The panel could fail to function if they have little experience of interviewing, and their questions might dry up.
- Members of the panel might be too aggressive towards the candidate or make him or her look 'silly'.

Exercise 21.3 First impressions

Why you should do this

To emphasise the importance of the first impressions that people make on others, and to give feedback to participants on how they 'come across'.

When to use this

On a one-to-one basis as a tutorial or in a workshop before participants have got to know each other.

What to do

If there are 12 people in the group, give each of them 11 pieces of paper with a pencil, some paper clips and a clipboard. Ask the participants to mingle and introduce themselves to each other in less than 2 minutes, describing what they do and saying at least one memorable thing about themselves. Each participant then writes down their first impressions of that person, both positive and negative (but not critical or insulting), puts the name of the individual concerned on the piece of paper (but not the name of the person making the comments), folds it, attaches a paper clip and gives it to the facilitator. These short exchanges and written impressions continue until everyone has introduced themselves to everyone else.

The facilitator sorts the comments and gives each participant those comments which relate to him or her. Each participant reads and absorbs all of the comments relating to them. The group finishes the session with a general discussion about the importance of first impressions and how accurate or otherwise these might be.

Whom to engage

This exercise works best with a dozen or so people, where the majority of individuals do not know one another.

How it works (insight)

It allows the participants to perceive how others see them.

How much time you should allow

Allow about 60 to 90 minutes for 12 people.

What the facilitator should do

The facilitator should provide pencils, paper, paper clips and clipboards as necessary. They should set ground rules to ensure that the feedback and comments are useful, covering positive and negative points but not being destructive or likely to cause distress.

What to do next

Individuals could use this feedback by discussing these comments with their mentor (if they have one) and comparing their own perceptions of the strengths and weaknesses of the impressions that they give. Then they might develop action plans to create the first impressions they wish to promote.

What makes it work better

Instead of people mingling together in a room, they could sit in a circle and introduce themselves in turn, describing their name and role and giving one or two memorable comments about themselves. The rest of the group could write down their perceptions of that person at the same time. These comments would then be collated by the facilitator and the exercise would move on to the next person.

What can go wrong

- Participants might be offended or distressed by some of the feedback, or expend energy trying to identify who made a particular comment.
- Meaningless or superficial comments might be made.

22

Making a presentation

Many people are frightened of giving a presentation or speaking in public. Every health professional or manager has to speak to groups of other people at some time, whether this is during a ward round, at a multidisciplinary case review or when presenting an interesting case at a postgraduate centre. If you want to be a teacher or to disseminate the results of a project, or lead and motivate others, you need to conquer this fear.

Good preparation should remove some of the anxiety. Think positively and prepare beforehand by imagining yourself giving the speech and everything going well. Try to exude an air of enthusiasm and confidence about the subject of your presentation.

The effectiveness of any speech will depend to a large extent on how much effort was put into preparing it. Be sure about the exact purpose of the presentation. Jot down your initial ideas in rough and add to them over time. Next organise them into a logical sequence and group your ideas under headings, and then expand each of the headings in a way that is appropriate to the target audience.

Help the audience to follow your train of thought and argument by setting out your talk as an introduction, a main theme in the body of the talk, and a final summary or conclusion. Let the audience know what to expect when you are introducing your presentation. 'Say what you are going to say, say it, and then repeat what you said', as is often recommended.

You should aim to start by capturing the interest of the audience, and then to maintain their attention and to finish with a memorable ending. Some opening gambits include the following:

* asking a rhetorical question
* repeating a quote or well-known saying
* reciting an anecdote
* telling a joke
* shocking your audience with an unexpected statement or a challenging remark
* making an emphatic statement or providing some facts.

Summarise your main messages. Finish with a well-polished relevant conclusion. This might be the answer to the rhetorical question posed at the beginning of the speech, the end of a story that was half told earlier in the presentation, or a challenge or action plan for the future. Do not simply tail off and stop abruptly, but make it clear that your talk has ended.

Some people write out their speeches in full, whilst others prefer to be prompted by notes prepared on cards with key headings. Fix your notes together with a treasury tag if they are on different cards or pages, so that you do not mix them up in your anxiety about speaking and if you do drop them they remain in order together. If you need to read the full text of the speech on the occasion, then make the size of the words large enough to be easily readable, and highlight the key points. Try to avoid simply reading out your presentation, and aim to talk *to* the audience rather than *at* them.

Practise your talk beforehand. Time it carefully and make sure that you leave enough time to dwell on the main points of interpretation and learning compared with the setting of the scene. Consider recording your practice talk and asking colleagues to comment on it constructively. Take off your watch and place it in a prominent position to remind you to keep to time – do not over-run or there will not be enough time for questions.

Develop your own style. Avoid trying to be funny if telling jokes makes you quake or you are hopeless at delivering the punchline. Do not be crude or swear in a professional setting. Have a glass of water available beside you if you are a nervous speaker.

Use of gestures

Your appearance and voice are vitally important, as well as what you say. Your gestures and body language should be in harmony with your voice and the messages of your presentation, and should not be distracting. Try and raise your eyes to scan the audience whenever you can remember to do so. Fix on one or two people when you are talking. Look up at the back rows to include them in your delivery, otherwise the learners sitting there will feel disconnected from the lecture.

Use your voice effectively

Make sure that you deliver your speech in such a way that your words are distinct. Try not to deliver the speech too quickly – even experienced speakers can fall into this trap.

Vary your tone and pitch in order to maintain interest. Your voice must be loud and clear enough to be heard by the people at the back of the audience. Change the pace of your presentation to add interest and variety to your talk. You might try for a dramatic effect occasionally by saying nothing and pausing for while.

Games, activities and learning techniques

Exercise 22.1 The restaurant review

Why you should do this

To understand how body language, tone and pitch of the voice, delivery and humour can affect the impact of a message on an audience. This should improve participants' presentation skills.

When to use this

Some time into a course, as this exercise requires a degree of confidence in public speaking.

What to do

1 Organise small groups of about six people (or at any rate an even number).
2 Divide the group into pairs and provide each individual with a script (e.g. a restaurant review from a Sunday newspaper).
3 Each participant picks one role from a list such as the following:
   • a vicar giving a sermon
   • a lawyer reading a statement outside a court
   • a newsreader on television or radio
   • someone who is very angry
   • someone who has their mind on other things
   • someone who is cynical
   • a member of parliament giving his or her maiden speech, etc.
4 Participants work in pairs for 10 to 15 minutes and practise their roles.
5 Each individual then has an opportunity to read the script in their role in front of the small group.
6 A discussion can then follow on the impact on the audience of the different styles and approaches used.

How it works (insight)

The same script is used by all of the participants, yet there are obvious differences in the delivery achieved through role play. The exercise allows participants to practise a range of presentation tools (e.g. body language, voice tone and pitch, speaking pace, eye contact, humour, etc.) in a friendly environment.

Whom to engage

This is a useful exercise for those who wish to improve their communication and presentation skills.

How much time you should allow

With a group of six people this exercise will take around an hour, allowing some time for discussion at the end.

What the facilitator should do

The facilitator should select a suitable article for the 'script'. Explain the sequence of this exercise and allow the participants time to select their roles.

What to do next

This could be a starting point for further communication and presentation skills exercises.

What makes it work better

- The script can be anything which takes two to three minutes to read. In practice, a relatively neutral article such as a review of a restaurant from a Sunday newspaper works better than a dramatic extract from a novel.
- The exercise should generate humour and entertain the participants.
- Depending on the level of experience of the participants, individuals could be allocated a role on a slip of paper and they could practise in pairs for 5 or 10 minutes and give each other feedback in an informal and friendly way before presenting to the larger group.

What can go wrong

Some participants may be nervous and find speaking in front of an audience traumatic.

Exercise 22.2 Sudden death: impromptu speaking

Why you should do this

To develop fast thinking, communication skills and courage in making presentations. It also develops an understanding of the importance of feedback, and the right and wrong ways to go about doing this.

When to use this

For participants who want to improve their communication skills and possibly leadership skills.

What to do

1   Introduce the participants to the essential elements of good public speaking and constructive feedback.
2   Select topics such as the following:
    *   my best holiday
    *   my favourite television programme when I was a child
    *   fictional/non-fictional heroes and heroines.
    Write these down on individual pieces of paper which are then folded and placed in a bowl.
3   Each participant picks a piece of paper from the bowl and addresses the audience and speaks for up to 2 minutes on the topic.
4   While the participant is giving their talk, the facilitator evaluates the speaker's performance. Once the first speaker has finished, the second speaker goes to the bowl, picks out a topic and then repeats the exercise, again for 2 minutes. This process is repeated until all of the participants have finished.
5   Feedback is given on each presentation to the whole workshop (e.g. as three or four positive points and one or two points for improvement).

How it works (insight)

The participant faces a friendly audience and receives positive and constructive feedback. This exercise also provides others with a practical demonstration of the skills that are required both in public speaking and in providing constructive feedback.

Whom to engage

Anyone who wants to improve their skills in making presentations.

How much time you should allow

Allow 10 minutes to explain the instructions. If there are 10 participants, then allow approximately 30 minutes to undertake each of the talks, and around 45 minutes for feedback and discussion.

What the facilitator should do

The facilitator should set up the room, list a number of topics on separate pieces of paper, and fold these and put them in the bowl. Recording sheets should include space for feedback on each person (e.g. confidence, posture, voice, and content and construction of the talk). The environment needs to be warm and friendly, and the speakers need to feel that they are being provided with constructive feedback in a non-threatening manner. The facilitator might use a stopwatch to ensure that the two-minute deadline is not exceeded.

What to do next

Concentrating on constructive feedback and subsequent discussion, these types of exercises could be repeated on a regular basis until improvements are seen. Often bad habits in public speaking are engrained, and it can take much practise to improve.

What makes it work better

- Instead of impromptu speaking, participants could speak for longer on a prepared topic.
- More than one person might critique the presentation, and the content and quality of their feedback could then be compared.
- An expert might be invited to join the session as a 'guest' evaluator, especially if the facilitator is not sufficiently experienced in public speaking.
- Ground rules might be set at the beginning that feedback should always be constructive.
- Participants might be advised that if they dry up and have nothing more to say they should finish the talk and return to their seats.

What can go wrong

- People can very easily dry up and have nothing to say. This can be embarrassing, and the person concerned could feel humiliated.
- Feedback might be too generalised to be helpful, or it might be too critical and thus damaging to the novice speakers.

Exercise 22.3 Bargains in the marketplace

Why you should do this

To improve creativity and skills such as persuasiveness and communication.

When to use this

In a workshop of around 10 people.

What to do

1　The facilitator brings along to the meeting a set of everyday objects such as cups, small trinkets, pens, books, photographs, etc. There need to be roughly twice as many objects as there are people in the group.
2　The objects are laid out on a large table and participants are asked to choose one object which they will have to persuade other members of the group to buy.
3　Individuals are divided into pairs on a random basis.
4　Each individual is asked to prepare a 2-minute talk to sell their particular object, and has 10 minutes to prepare their presentation. Their partner acts as a coach whose role is to provide ideas and feedback and to help the individual to prepare their talk. After 10 minutes the roles are reversed and the person who prepared the talk now acts as the coach.
5　Each of the pairs has a stall, and all members of the workshop gather round each stall in turn where individuals have up to 2 minutes to persuade other members of the workshop to buy their particular item.
6　The workshop then moves on to the next stall, etc., until all of the participants have had an opportunity to sell their individual item.
7　Finally, all of the participants select the item(s) they wish to buy.

You could dispense with a coach in this exercise if you prefer, and let individuals work on their presentations by themselves.

How it works (insight)

This exercise allows the participants to experiment with different styles of persuasion – especially if such an approach does not come naturally.

Whom to engage

Any learners might benefit from this exercise.

How much time you should allow

Allow about 10 minutes for explaining the purpose of the exercise and for individuals to select items, 20 minutes to prepare their speeches, and another 30 minutes for allowing each participant to have an opportunity to sell their item.

What the facilitator should do

Provide various items that will stimulate interest, and lay them out on a table large enough for the participants to mingle around. Keep people to time, particularly when making their sales pitch in their market stalls within the 2-minute time limit.

What to do next

The group may discuss how the session went and identify what tempted people to buy certain items. How were people persuaded? What role did the coach play? What makes a good coach?

Each coach could provide feedback to his or her partner.

What makes it work better

The selection of items is important, and unusual objects could be selected in order to stimulate creative presentations.

What can go wrong

Participants who are not comfortable about speaking in public may find the exercise threatening.

23

Written and audiovisual aids to learning

A good teacher delivers education at a level, in a style and at a time that is most appropriate to the learner – when the latter is ready and will gain most benefit. Such a teacher will also need a variety of props and aids to help them to convey the information that they want the learner to hear, understand and apply at work.

Use the most appropriate audiovisual aids to command your audience's attention. However, do not be totally reliant on your audiovisual equipment, in case there is a technical hitch and you have to perform unaided.

Writing: handouts, reports

The rules for effective writing for you as a teacher or for your learners can be summarised as follows.

- Write in clear, simple language.
- Use short sentences.
- Do not use two-syllable words if there is a one-syllable option.
- Pitch the content at the right level for the reader.
- Make the layout attractive, with plenty of white space.
- Include boxes for key points.
- Use subheadings to break up the text.
- Add illustrations and diagrams to complement the text.
- Focus on relevant material rather than on rambling anecdotes.
- Explain any jargon or abbreviations.

A handout should capture the key points of your talk, but need not be too comprehensive, as those who are particularly interested in the topic can follow up your session with private reading. Include a reading list or references to key literature or sources of further information. Always remember to credit other people's work, giving full references.

PowerPoint presentations

You can read up on the tips for 'effective PowerPoint presentations for the technologically challenged' described by Holzl,[1] which give practical advice that includes story boarding, size of fonts, use of colour and common pitfalls. The key points are as follows.

1 Choose a format for your presentation that is in keeping with the theme of your talk.
2 Use clear legible text in short phrases or sentences.
3 Match the font size to the size of the lecture room (e.g. a 36-point-size text in lecture theatres with more than 200 seats, or a 24-point-size text in rooms with less than 50 seats).
4 Include a maximum of one idea per screen.
5 Limit yourself to six or fewer words per line in six or less lines.
6 Predominantly lower-case letters are more comprehensible than CAPITALS.
7 Maximise the contrast between text and background.
8 Build your PowerPoint slides into a logical sequence for the presentation.
9 Take along a duplicate set of slides for overhead projection as a safeguard in case the PowerPoint equipment does not work on the day.

Overhead projection slides

This technique involves a similar approach to that for PowerPoint presentations. Consider using a cellophane film enclosure for your overheads so that they fit within an A4 cardboard file, keeping them in order and protected from the clutter of your everyday life.

A logo in one corner gives the impression of a coherent set of slides. Scan a picture on to an overhead transparency film, from your PC. Consider investing in a digital camera for capturing unusual photographs to illustrate your talk in an original way.

Video film

Showing a video can disrupt the flow of your presentation. If you do show one, explain the points that you want to bring out before you show it, and then after the viewers have finished watching it expand on what they will have noticed. Keep the video film short in order to maintain the momentum of the presentation.

Any patient who appears on an educational video must have given their informed consent to be filmed and know the context in which you will be using and showing the video.

Using a flip chart

A flip chart is a useful interactive educational tool unless the person writing on it stands with their back to everyone else, blocking the view and listing their own ideas. Use a flip chart for brainstorming and problem solving to capture everyone's ideas. Then display the completed sheets around the walls of the room for easy reference.

Always carry a flip-chart pen in your bag. You never know when you are at a meeting whether it will unexpectedly be useful to be able to capture the ideas in a discussion on a flip chart or whiteboard.

Much of the material in this section is derived from Chambers R and Wall D (2000) *Teaching Made Easy*. Radcliffe Medical Press, Oxford.

Reference

1   Holzl J (1997) Twelve tips for effective PowerPoint presentations for the technologically challenged. *Med Teacher*. **19**: 175–9.

Games, activities and learning techniques

Exercise 23.1 Using an active photograph

Why you should use this

To stimulate discussion and trigger lateral thinking when looking at a topic in depth for new solutions or innovations.

When to use this

Early on in small group work it can help the participants to start talking and the group to begin to gel. Later on in small or large group work it can waken up a fatigued audience by changing the pace and style of the learning event and introducing new ideas.

What to do

Select a photograph that is relevant to the theme of the learning event. Invite the participants to discuss the issues portrayed by the photograph, first in general and then in depth in a semi-structured format, responding to questions that you pose. For instance, the right photograph might trigger general and then in-depth discussions about the health issues illustrated, the societal and environmental factors that are likely to be associated with the pictures, and alternative interventions that could be tried to tackle those health issues.

Discuss in small groups with subsequent feedback in a plenary group.

How it works (insight)

The visual imagery will appeal to everyone and prove the saying 'a picture is worth a thousand words'.

Whom to engage

Everyone should be engaged by the right photograph. You can expect previously disinterested or non-contributing members of the group to become engaged in discussion.

How much time you should allow

The time allowed will depend on the complexity of the scene in the photograph (e.g. how many clues there are to spot that are not initially obvious) and the number and type of questions that you pose for debate. As the exercise progresses, the photograph itself will become less important and the group discussion will be what absorbs the participants. The exercise will probably take a minimum of 30 minutes in most instances for the group work, followed by a minimum of 15 minutes for feedback to the facilitator.

What the facilitator should do

Choose the right photograph for the exercise, which is relevant to the theme of the learning event and that depicts problem issues for which the participants can discuss solutions. Divide the participants into groups of no more than 10 people so that everyone can see and perhaps handle a copy of the photograph. Pose challenging questions for debate, and encourage the group to appoint a spokesperson who can report back afterwards in the plenary feedback session. Encourage successive spokespeople from different small groups to contribute new points only. Rotate the spokesperson to start giving feedback for each question posed for debate.

What to do next

Make action plans in small groups or pairs to think out the proposed solutions in more detail. The timetabled action plan should include the implementation of the solution and subsequent evaluation of the change.

What makes it work better

- A photograph portraying a variety of activities or drama, giving plenty of material for discussion.
- Enough copies of a reasonable-sized photograph (e.g. at least 8 by 12 inches) so that everyone can easily observe the fine points of the picture. It does not matter whether it is a black-and-white or coloured photograph, so photocopies will be fine so long as the reproduction is sharp.
- You can substitute a reasonable-sized painting for the photograph if the number of participants is small enough to be able to work from one image.

What can go wrong

- You may choose the wrong photograph, which portrays something relevant to the topic of the learning event to you, but to few of the participants.
- You may not explain the task properly or set the most appropriate framework for discussion of the issues depicted in the photograph, so that it does not serve as a trigger for discussion.
- Similarly, the scene in the photograph might be too simple to act as a challenging stimulus for debate.

Exercise 23.2 Adding a subtitle to a cartoon or completing a thoughts/speech bubble

Why you should use this

To inject humour into a teaching session.

When to use this

You could use this exercise in a workshop or a succession of plenary lectures in a day's course to:

- liven up the meeting
- encourage collaboration
- provide a different style of learning to appeal to activists

- give the teacher a 'rest' from talking and the audience a rest from the teacher.

What to do

Select a cartoon that has no title and invite the participants to think of an appropriate heading. Alternatively, choose a cartoon or picture of one or more people doing something or thinking something, and then draw in one or more speech bubbles for the participants to fill in. The essence of the cartoon should be relevant to the theme of your learning event. Ask the participants to work on the task in pairs or small groups.

You could ask the participants to report back by calling out their contributions, writing their suggestions on the cartoon and pinning them up on a board for participants to look at at their leisure, or writing their responses on 'post-it' notes and sticking these up beneath a replica of the cartoon for general inspection.

How it works (insight)

Working with others will generate more ideas and humour as suggestions are exchanged and these become more outrageous. It will lighten the atmosphere and put everyone in a good mood for subsequent learning sessions.

Whom to engage

Anyone and everyone.

How much time you should allow

Allow up to 15 minutes, according to how the interchange and laughter are going.

What the facilitator should do

Choose a cartoon or a person/group of people in the scene that is likely to trigger ideas and amusement.

What to do next

Try the same exercise with another cartoon and another group of learners, in order to find out by experience which pictures provoke the most useful discussion or laughter, with whom and when.

What makes it work better

You could offer a prize for the best 'answer'. Invite the participants to vote for the one they like best by appending a coloured dot to the displayed responses or ticking a chart that lists the suggestions.

What can go wrong

Individual participants might wander off to make calls on their mobile phones because they consider this exercise to be one they can miss out.

24

Learning about evidence-based practice: protocols, guidelines and patient group directives

Protocols

Protocols have come to have a specific meaning within the health service. The purpose of a protocol is to direct healthcare staff along preferred pathways by outlining detailed management plans for discrete (usually clinical) conditions. These conditions are judged to be suitable for stepwise decision-making processes that can be specified in flow diagrams or algorithms.[1] Protocols are considered to be more restrictive than guidelines, and their relevance to clinical situations is limited to certain specific occasions when their rigidity of purpose minimises risk. They are often used when treatment is delegated to staff who would not otherwise have this responsibility and who do not have the knowledge or training to deviate from the protocol.

Guidelines

Guidelines are a collection of recommendations that embody certain standards of management. These standards are (or should be) based on evidence and may:

- set out minimum reasonable standards
- codify customary standards
- recommend best practice.

Recommendations

Recommendations are usually less strongly worded than guidelines, and may be based on less certain evidence. Sometimes they are used almost interchangeably with guidelines, but they often imply recommended action suggested by an expert (or committee of experts) to non-experts.

Codes of practice

Codes of practice usually relay not only guidelines on safety and efficacy, but also ethical and social aspects of the problems.

Practice or workplace policies

Practice policies consist of agreed courses of action (or guidelines) in specific clinical or non-clinical situations. They direct the healthcare staff to take certain actions for groups of patients or for individuals. They tend to be reached by consensus after discussion of various options, considering the consequences of those options and then deciding on the desirability of particular outcomes for patients.[2]

Patient group directives

These are used to authorise health professionals without prescribing authority (e.g. practice nurses) to supply or administer prescription-only medicines to patients who are not seen first by a doctor. The Medicines Act allows only doctors, dentists and veterinary practitioners to prescribe prescription-only medicines, but others can administer them with written or verbal instructions. The Medicines Act was amended in 2000 to allow patient group directives to be used by specified health professionals.[3] There are certain criteria that must be included in the directive, so consult the legal requirements when drawing them up. The clinical staff who will be involved in using the group directive should be consulted with regard to its construction and application. A useful website that gives guidance on protocols and group directives is www.groupprotocols.org.uk, and the Royal College of Nursing have detailed guidance on their website, www.rcn.org.uk/professional/professional_nursing issues_patientgroup_when.html.

The evidence for protocols and guidelines[4-7]

There are several systems of grading evidence. A classification[4] that is often quoted gives the strength of evidence as shown in Box 24.1.

Box 24.1: Strength of evidence

Type I: Strong evidence from at least one systematic review of multiple well-designed randomised controlled trials (RCTs)

Type II: Strong evidence from at least one properly designed randomised controlled trial of appropriate size

Type III: Evidence from well-designed trials without randomisation, single group pre–post, cohort, time-series or matched case–control studies

Type IV: Evidence from well-designed non-experimental studies from more than one centre or research group

Type V: Opinions of respected authorities, based on clinical evidence, descriptive studies or reports of expert committees

---

Other categories of evidence[5] are listed in the compendium of the best available evidence for effective healthcare – *Clinical Evidence* – which is updated every six months, and is perhaps more useful to the health professional in everyday work. Box 24.2 describes these categories.

Box 24.2: Categories of evidence

Beneficial: Interventions whose effectiveness has been shown by clear evidence from controlled trials

Likely to be beneficial: Interventions whose effectiveness is less well established than for those listed under 'beneficial'

Trade-off between benefits and harm: Interventions for which clinicians and patients should weigh up the beneficial and harmful effects according to individual circumstances and priorities

Unknown effectiveness: Interventions for which there are currently insufficient data, or data of inadequate quality (this includes interventions that are widely accepted as beneficial but which have never been formally tested in randomised controlled trials, often because the latter would be regarded as unethical)

Unlikely to be beneficial: Interventions for which lack of effectiveness is less well established than for those listed under 'likely to be ineffective or harmful'

Likely to be ineffective or harmful: Interventions whose ineffectiveness or harmfulness has been demonstrated by clear evidence

---

Using guidelines

The key features determining whether local guidelines worked in one initiative[8] were as follows.

- There was multidisciplinary involvement in drawing them up.
- A well-described systematic review of the literature underpinned the guidelines, with graded recommendations for best practice linked to the evidence.
- Ownership was nurtured at national and local levels.
- A local implementation plan ensured that all of the practicalities (time, staff, education and training, resources) were foreseen and met, stakeholders were supported and predictors of sustainability were addressed (guideline usability, individualising guidelines to practitioners and patients).

References

1 Schoenbaum S and Gottlieb L (1990) Algorithm-based improvement of clinical quality. *BMJ.* **301**: 1374–6.

2 Hurwitz B (1998) *Clinical Guidelines and the Law*. Radcliffe Medical Press, Oxford.

3 National Health Service Executive (2000) *Patient Group Directives (England)*. Department of Health, London.

4 Muir Gray JA (1997) *Evidence-Based Healthcare*. Churchill Livingstone, Edinburgh.

5 Barton S (ed.) (2001) *Clinical Evidence. Issue 5*. BMJ Publishing Group, London.

6 Sackett D, Richardson WS, Rosenberg W and Haynes RB (1997) *Evidence-Based Medicine. How to practise and teach EBM*. Churchill Livingstone, London.

7 Straus SE, Badenoch D, Richardson WS *et al.* (1998) *Practising Evidence-Based Medicine: learner's manual* (3e). Radcliffe Medical Press, Oxford.

8 Donald P (2000) Promoting the local ownership of guidelines. *Guidelines Pract.* **3**: 17.

Games, activities and learning techniques

Exercise 24.1 The simplest task is complicated

Why you should do this

This exercise demonstrates how difficult it is to write down every action that should be carried out, and to decide who does what.

When to use this

Either when people are first starting to write protocols, etc., or when they think that they know how to do this, but are inexperienced in their application.

What to do

Set a scenario that is familiar and which can be challenged by unexpected happenings (*see* the scenario suggestions below). Divide the group into syndicate groups; six to eight people in a group is an ideal size for creating some diversity but not too much. Each group writes a protocol for the scenario. In the plenary session each syndicate group presents their protocol. After all of these have been presented, allow time for discussion of the differences and similarities, and for correction of any deficiencies. Then ask the groups to think up some pitfalls, some aspects that could make the protocols unworkable, and write one or two on each flip-chart protocol. Add your own suggestions if there are not enough. Each syndicate group then takes away their own protocol and modifies it to accommodate the pitfall(s). Finally, they return to the plenary session and present the modified version.

How it works (insight)

It becomes apparent how difficult it is to write a protocol for what seem to be simple tasks. The problems that are unforeseen can make it impossible – the participants realise that there has to be a failsafe of independent action.

Whom to engage

People who are fairly new to the idea of either writing or using protocols, or those whom you have identified as being over-confident about initiating and designing tools!

How much time you should allow

Allow 10 minutes for explaining the task, setting the scenario and dividing into groups. Allow 40 minutes for drawing up and writing the protocol, 5 minutes each for presenting it and 20 minutes for general discussion. Then allocate 10 minutes for thinking up pitfalls and another 15 minutes for modifications. The participants should need only 2 to 3 minutes to present the modifications, if they have managed any. Allow a further 20 minutes for general discussion, and then summarise the conclusions. Thus the exercise will take over 2 hours in total.

What the facilitator should do

Prepare the scenarios. Possible scenarios could include preparing to leave on holiday in a caravan with a dog, washing up at a scout camp, or obtaining travel insurance for a family holiday abroad. Think up some problems that might occur to make these tasks more complicated or require modification (e.g. the dog runs off, there is a thunderstorm at the scout camp, an aged aunt wants to go on holiday with them). You will need at least one problem per syndicate group.

Keep the exercise light-hearted, keep it moving fairly fast, keep to time and be prepared to bring people back to the plenary group earlier if they are looking frustrated or bored. Summarise some general conclusions.

What to do next

Discuss how the general conclusions could be used in the participants' workplace before moving on to further work or a different subject.

What makes it work better

- Imaginative solutions and a sense of fun, with participants entering into the spirit of the game.
- You could provide a 'lucky dip' of problems that are generally applicable to most situations. For example:
  1 a thunderstorm causes a torrential downpour and affects phones and electricity supplies
  2 someone is suddenly taken ill
  3 your party is involved in an outbreak of an infectious disease
  4 one or two key people are unavailable
  5 a fuel blockade prevents you from obtaining fuel
  6 a burglar steals essential equipment.

What can go wrong

Participants may take the exercise too seriously, or conversely consider it too trivial to bother with.

Exercise 24.2   All change

Why you should do this

This exercise helps people who have little or no experience of writing guidelines, etc., to understand the procedure better.

When to use this

With a group that is going to have to draw up guidelines or patient group directives, etc.

What to do

Provide quite a number of protocols, patient group directives, guidelines, etc., as handouts. It is helpful to include several on the same subject if you can find them, and clip them together. Divide the group into syndicate groups of four to six people, and try to mix levels of experience if possible (you may need to establish this from the participants first).

Divide the pile of prepared handouts into roughly equal heaps for each syndicate group. Ask them to sort through them and select one or two to revise. The syndicate group then tries to revise the handout so that it is suitable for use in their own working environment. Ask them to record any variations that might be needed in each individual's workplace. They should record their revised document on flip-chart sheets.

In the plenary session when all of the participants come together, each syndicate group should present their own document and explain briefly the reasons behind any variation. Allow a short time for discussion of each.

How it works (insight)

This exercise helps people who are starting to look at drawing up such documents to understand how they need to be tailored for their own use. They understand that there is not just 'one way' of doing it, and that they need to choose suitable instruments for their own environment.

Whom to engage

The exercise is very useful for beginners.

How much time you should allow

Allow about 45 minutes for the modifications (and less if they are more experienced, to put the pressure on!). Give the presenter from each syndicate group 8 minutes to present and explain, and allow about 15 minutes of discussion time for each. Then allow time for a general discussion, noting any general points on the flip chart.

What the facilitator should do

You need plenty of documents so that the participants have to make a choice. For complete beginners you may need to give some illustrations of what might need changing, in which case prepare some examples of your own, not using the ones that you have copied.

Keep time, and encourage contributions and constructive praise and criticism in the plenary session.

What to do next

Offer to have the participants' own flip-chart documents typed up and sent to them. Offer to let them take away the copied documents for future work.

What makes it work better

- Groups who are not too disparate with regard to their knowledge and skills.
- Guidelines or directives that apply to more than one professional or staff group.

What can go wrong

- Participants may have very different levels of knowledge and skills.
- Guidelines or directives may only apply to some of the group members, so that the others cannot see the relevance of them, or feel that they cannot contribute.

Exercise 24.3   Guideline subversives

Why you should do this

This exercise illustrates some of the difficulties involved in drawing up protocols or guidelines.

When to use this

If the participants need to improve their skills or appreciate the difficulties involved in drawing up guidelines.

What to do

Ask the participants to bring a task from their workplace for which a protocol or guideline is required. The facilitator should be aware of the type of guidelines that might be applicable to the participants' work, and be prepared with some ideas in case the group members bring few examples. Bring enough copies of the legal requirements for patient group directives for each person to have one as a reference.

Write down on a flip chart what the participants have brought (you may have enough without your ideas). You may find that some are very similar and can be grouped together. Discard any that are too complex. Ask the participants to assign themselves to a subject. You may find that one or two people are on their own, so negotiate with them what they want to do. Encourage them to learn about the process by working on another subject with others. Try to keep the group size to about four to five people per subject.

Each group takes one subject and draws up a guideline or protocol with a nominated or volunteered person as the scribe. After a break, each scribe takes the guideline or protocol to another group. The new group takes each part of the guideline or protocol in turn and suggests ways in which it could be subverted. The scribe writes on the comments using a pen of another colour.

The participants then reconvene in a plenary group, and each scribe presents the guideline or protocol together with the subversive comments. The facilitator writes up the types of subversive behaviour described and classifies their behaviour into types of problems that might be encountered.

How it works (insight)

Presenting a guideline or protocol for subversion can liberate people to be quite destructive, but it also allows them to appreciate how difficult it can be to implement guidelines or protocols without the full collaboration and support of all involved.

Whom to engage

Any group that wishes to improve their skills in guideline or protocol development.

How much time you should allow

You will need about 30 minutes to write up the tasks and divide into groups. Allow an hour for writing the guideline or protocol, have a break for at least 20 minutes, and then allow 30 to 40 minutes for the subversion. The plenary group feedback usually takes about 30 to 45 minutes. If the group is very inexperienced, you may want to have longer (1½ hours) for the guideline or protocol writing, and then break for lunch before the subversion.

What the facilitator should do

Keep the groups to time so that they all finish together. You will need to encourage them to write down the protocol or guideline – they usually spend most of the time talking about it, so warn them at least 10 minutes before the end. Keep the atmosphere light-hearted.

What to do next

The group may want to move on to more serious planning for work on a task that can be completed.

What makes it work better

A light-hearted atmosphere and participants who have some experience of writing and using protocols and guidelines.

What can go wrong

- Some of the participants may be subordinate to others in the group in an organisation that is autocratic. They will then take the task too seriously and be unable to be creative in their subversive activities.
- People may be too possessive about their own protocol or guideline and become upset when the other group points out the areas where it might be undermined.

25

Endpiece

Adult learning has become essential in this modern, changing and complex world. Relying on our initial education and training is totally inadequate for the rest of our working lives. Non-participation in adult learning automatically disadvantages certain individuals or groups as they fall behind their peers.

Increasing the choice in *how* people learn is saying to the learners and facilitators that there are these particular things that we need to find out about, or to know how to do, and there are these two or three different ways of doing it. As well, learners require assistance so that they can identify *what* it is that they need to learn about.

Most adult learners prefer to learn in groups. Even when they use 'self-directed learning' such as reading, distance learning packages, or practising a skill, they still want to get together to discuss and bounce ideas off each other or compare techniques. The learning group can often achieve more for the individual group members together than can be achieved alone. The group may provide a challenge for learners, support them while they change and learn, and provide alternative ways of thinking or functioning.

Remember that learning is still an individual activity; the personal change required has to be achieved alone, however helpful the group can be. A group can inhibit change in individuals by exerting pressure on them to conform or adopt one particular role. The pace of a group may be too slow or too fast. Learning, and change, must take place outside group activities as well. This book has not included much on techniques of one-to-one learning from mentors, supervisors or peers, but these must not be forgotten as important additional techniques. Self-directed instruction always has a major part to play in any acquisition of knowledge, skill or alteration of attitudes. Life-long learning is learning about how best to learn, and like finding out how to use a library, and how to look things up, it stays with you for ever.

Index